DIABETIC'S GUIDE
to Health and Fitness

An Authoritative Approach to Leading an Active Life

KRIS E. BERG, EdD
University of Nebraska at Omaha

Leisure Press
Champaign, Illinois

Library of Congress Cataloging-in-Publication Data

Berg, Kris E., 1943-
   Diabetic's guide to health and fitness / by Kris E. Berg.
      p.   cm.
   Reprint. Originally published: Champaign, Ill. : Life Enhancement
Publications, 1986.
   Includes bibliographical references and index.
   ISBN 0-88011-347-2
   1. Diabetes--Exercise therapy.   2. Diabetes--Popular works.
3. Diabetics--Health and hygiene.   4. Physical fitness.   I. Title.
RC661.E94B47   1991
616.4'62--dc20
                                                         91-408
                                                         CIP

Copyright © 1986 by Kris E. Berg

ISBN: 0-88011-347-2
(Previously published by Life Enhancement Publications,
ISBN 0-87322-901-0)

Developmental Editor: Sue Ingels Mauck
Copy Editor: Ann Morris Bruehler
Production Director: Ernie Noa
Typesetter: Theresa Bear
Text Design: Julie Szamocki
Text Layout: Lezli Harris
Cover Design and Layout: Jack Davis
Cover Photo: Index Stock International Inc.
Photos in text: Tim Fitzgerald
Printed By: Phillips Brothers, Inc.

Printed in the United States of America

10   9   8   7   6   5   4

Leisure Press
A Division of Human Kinetics
   Publishers
Box 5076, Champaign, IL
61825-5076
1-800-747-4457

Canada Office:
Human Kinetics Publishers
P.O. Box 2503, Windsor, ON
N8Y 4S2
1-800-465-7301 (in Canada only)

Europe Office:
Human Kinetics Publishers (Europ
   Ltd.
P.O. Box IW14
Leeds LS16 6TR
England
0532-781708

Australia Office:
Human Kinetics Publishers
P.O. Box 80
Kingswood 5062
South Australia
374-0433

Contents

Introduction   vii
Acknowledgments   x

Part I: The Basics   1

chapter 1: The Sad Side of the Story   3

chapter 2: Good News for Diabetics   7

    Exercise and Diabetic Management   8
    Weight Loss and Control   9
    Muscular Fitness   10
    Reduced Need for Medication or Insulin   11
    Improved Self-Image   12
    Coping With Stress   12

chapter 3: Components of Good Diabetic Control 15

    Blood Sugar Assessment   18
    Consistency   21
    Multiple Daily Insulin Injections   21
    Correction Plan   24

Part II: Physical Fitness   27

chapter 4: Special Concerns for Exercising   29
Diabetics

Energy Cost of Various Activities   29
Energy Sources During Exercise   32
The Effect of Exercise on Insulin Requirement   35
Planning Ahead for Exercise   36
The Effects of Insulin on the Capacity to Exercise   37
Injection Site   38
The Day After Extensive Exercise   39
Summary   39

chapter 5: Principles of Exercise   41

Consult Your Physician   41
Start Comfortably   42
Warm-Up and Cool-Down   45
Consistency   47
Total Fitness   48
Progression   48

chapter 6: Aerobic Fitness   49

Intensity   50
Duration   56
Frequency   56
Mode   57
Other Considerations   58

chapter 7: Muscular Fitness   67

Importance of Muscular Fitness   67
Training Principles   68
Basic Strength Exercises   78

chapter 8: Flexibility   97

   Testing and Developing Your Flexibility   99
   How to Stretch   111

chapter 9: Weight Control   115

   Disadvantages of Obesity   116
   Societal Standards   118
   Women and Weight Control   121
   Do We Even Need Fat in Our Bodies?   122
   How Much Fat Is too Much?   122
   What Causes Obesity?   124
   The Role of Exercise in Weight Control   126
   Dietary Aspects of Weight Control   139

Part III: Putting It All Together   163

chapter 10: Adapting to Stress   165

   What Is Stress?   166
   The American Work Ethic and Stress   169
   How Do I Start?   172
   Learning to Say "No"   172
   Symptoms of Stress   174
   Coping Techniques   175
   Effect of Diet and Drugs on Stress   185
   Coping on the Move   190
   Work Efficiency and Stress   191
   A Philosophy of Life to Reduce Stress   196
   Summary   197

chapter 11: Handling Special and Unexpected   199
   Conditions

   Illness   199
   Surgery   200

Pregnancy   201
Medications   202
Stress   203
Identification   204
Snack Food While Traveling   204
Emergency Supplies in the Car   204
Delayed Meals   205
Eating Out   205
Treating Insulin Reaction   206
Treating an Insulin Reaction in Public   207
Treating Ketoacidosis   208
Prolonged Inactivity   209
Prolonged Physical Activity   210
On the Job   215
Staying on Schedule with Insulin and Oral   215
    Medication
Holidays   216

chapter 12: Motivation   219

Principles of Motivation   220
Analysis of Factors That Affect Behavior   224
The Ascending Health Spiral   227
A Theory of Health Behavior   228
Tips on Eating for Weight Control   229
Tips on Developing an Exercise Habit   234
Motivating and Helping the Young Diabetic   245

appendix A: Additional Reading   247

appendix B: Diabetic Organizations and   251
    Community Resources

References   255

Index   257

Introduction

I was first diagnosed as an insulin-dependent diabetic at age 12. The year was 1955. I remember measuring urine glucose by chemical analysis. That procedure involved placing a urine specimen in a test tube with a blue-colored liquid called Benedict's solution. The mixture was boiled for several minutes and then the color was assessed, which provided only a "guesstimate" of my blood sugar. This procedure was done four times a day and included obtaining a urine specimen at school prior to lunch. You can imagine the fun a 12-year-old junior high school student had doing that. I also remember boiling my syringe and needle each morning for 5 minutes to sterilize them. The point I want to make is that these procedures took considerable time and compared to today's technology, they were less valid and accurate.

How times have changed; so much has been learned in the past several decades. We can now measure blood sugar easily at home instead of having to take periodic tests at the doctor's office or relying on the less accurate urine measurements. Disposable syringes/needles are used almost exclusively. The needles of today have a smaller diameter and no burrs or rough edges. Consequently, they are nearly painless. Many of us use multiple daily insulin injections to attain more stable blood sugar levels, whereas years ago most people with type I diabetes took only one injection each day. With such advances, it appears that the major stumbling block today for people with diabetes is simply not making use of these improvements.

While writing this book at age 41, 29 years after being diagnosed as a diabetic, I realize how fortunate I am. The physician who first treated me was a firm but positive man.

Perhaps knowing I was a very physically active young boy made him approach me differently. He told me about Bill Talbert, a Davis Cup tennis player, who was diabetic. Other comments about my diabetic management resulted in my belief that I could continue doing all the things I had been doing. To me, that meant life was going to be okay. Having lost considerable weight and muscle in the several months prior to diagnosis, I was eager to build myself up physically. While in the hospital and being placed on insulin, I began a regimen of push-ups, other calisthenics, and running in place. That simple program established an exercise habit that assisted me in playing sports in high school and college, competing in AAU Olympic weight lifting and power lifting, completing a decathlon, and running a marathon. I still enjoy the thrill of training and competing and I participate in long-distance running and intramural basketball at the university where I teach, and I cross-country ski and backpack whenever possible. Not so strangely, I received my doctorate in exercise physiology. My teaching and research career allows me the opportunity to help others improve their lives via appropriate exercise, diet, and overall health care.

One of my younger brothers became diabetic at age 8. He died of diabetic complications at age 30. His last several years were greatly limited by blindness and kidney disease that necessitated dialysis and kidney transplant. He never fully adapted to the insulin-diet-activity regimen that the diabetic condition demands and he suffered the consequences. In memory of my brother, this book is addressed foremost to persons with diabetes, each of whom is almost solely accountable for his or her state of health, and secondly to family members and friends who can offer support and gain insights into what diabetic individuals are trying to accomplish. It should be realized from the onset that the key premise of this book is that each diabetic must know his or her unique condition extremely well. Optimal diabetic control requires a constant effort to adjust insulin, food, and physical activity to achieve a normal blood sugar level for as much of the time as possible. It should be good news that diabetic management does make a big difference in how you feel emotionally and physically, and on your overall health status. Many of the dietary and exercise guidelines described here apply to nondiabetics as well. Diabetics would do well to realize that the optimal diabetic lifestyle could well serve as a model for most people. Consequently, being a "good" diabetic isn't as unique as one might think. Today's emphasis on health promotion and healthy lifestyle means that the special things we do to control our blood sugar are in vogue. Eating fruit for dessert, avoiding fatty foods, and drinking diet beverages are typical eating patterns today.

Many people with diabetes are sensitive to being called a "diabetic." I understand why but I also feel it is awkward and cumbersome to use the word only as an adjective (such as "diabetic persons") or as a noun in reference to a disease rather than a person (such as "people with diabetes"). I have attempted to use appropriate terminology in many instances but in some places it seemed to make the reading lengthy and laborious. From my personal standpoint, I view my life as one in which I am a diabetic. I eat as a diabetic, exercise as a diabetic, and travel as a diabetic. In short, I examine the effects of nearly everything I do on my diabetic well-being. To do less defies being well-regulated and healthy. So, I apologize beforehand to those who may feel offended. I use the terms knowingly.

The long-range goal of this book is to help people with diabetes maximize what can be accomplished in their lives by using today's technology and knowledge. While medical miracles are developing, they should not detract from diabetics' sense of responsibility in regulating the control of their condition. It is this sense of lifelong and daily commitment that I have noted lacking in too many people with diabetes. So, eat like an Olympic athlete, exercise like a Hollywood star or starlet, take insulin or oral medication on a basis to keep your blood sugar near optimum, and measure your blood sugar to determine the degree to which the total system is in balance. Your discipline and efforts will pay dividends on an hourly, daily, and lifetime basis. Your life is not a bad investment.

Acknowledgments

The time spent writing this book is impressive. I thank my wife, Carolyn, for her strong encouragement to write the book and her support throughout, and my two sons, Eric and Steve, for playing ball with me, which provided a marvelous break from writing. I thank my parents for their love and motivation over the years, and calm assurance when I was a boy that I could cope with having diabetes. I thank Marilyn R. Adams for the quality job in typing, proofing, and making editorial suggestions. Lastly, I thank Tim Fitzgerald for taking the photographs that appear in this book.

part I

The Basics

chapter 1

The Sad Side of the Story

Medical and health statistics concerning diabetics are quite frightening. Diabetics as a group are at increased risk for a number of disease states such as cardiovascular disease, eye problems, nerve disorders and kidney failure. What is more, diabetes is currently the fifth leading cause of death in the United States and third if complications of the condition are included. While the exact cause or causes of diabetic complications are not fully understood, the underlying factor that appears to make those with diabetes more prone to so many health problems is prolonged and frequent elevation of blood sugar. Some of the excess sugar or glucose accumulates in various tissues, thereby reducing their function. For example, excess glucose in the blood damages the walls of the capillaries, the smallest type of blood vessel in the body. The passage of nutrients such as glucose, fats, and amino acids as well as oxygen is impaired with such damage. Consequently, the tissues supplied by damaged capillaries gradually decrease in function. Some people with diabetes suffer infection or amputation of limbs where circulation is greatly impaired.

Damaged nerves don't transmit nerve impulses as well as healthy nerves do; this can lead to impotency, reduced muscle function, and even loss of pain sensitivity. Many diabetics have so little feeling in their toes and feet, for example, that they may not even be aware of injuries to their feet. Because of the reduced local blood circulation, healing of an injury is considerably slower in people with diabetes. The hands and feet are frequently found to be uncomfortably cold even when the rest of the body is warm.

The filtering mechanism of the kidneys is impaired in many people with diabetes. Normal kidney function decreases, and many substances in the blood (e.g., proteins and enzymes) rise to unusually high levels. This is one reason why your physician has you collect a urine specimen with each visit: to assess the function of your kidneys by examining the level of such substances in your urine. Urinary infections are also more common in diabetics because high blood glucose levels encourage bacterial growth.

The eyes also undergo changes as vessel damage occurs. Glucose enters the lens and combines with chemicals to produce cataracts. Diabetic retinopathy (or damaged retina) results from damage to the blood vessels supplying the retina. The vessels balloon, finally rupture, and allow bleeding within the eye. Light entering the eye and passing through the orbit on its way to the retina is blocked and vision is impaired. However, recent evidence indicates that this damage can be halted and even partially reversed with good blood sugar control.

Heart and blood vessel problems are two to three times more frequent in people with diabetes. They possess more risk factors including obesity (people with adult-onset diabetes or type 2 diabetes are typically overweight), elevated blood fats such as cholesterol and triglyceride, elevated blood pressure, increased blood clotting tendency and reduced dissolving of blood clots, and low levels of aerobic or cardiorespiratory fitness. These blood and blood vessel changes are accompanied by a reduced quantity of oxygen carried by the blood. Also, less oxygen is released by the blood to the tissues when diabetes is poorly controlled, because the chemical composition of hemoglobin, the molecule that carries the oxygen, is altered by the prolonged elevation of blood glucose. High glucose concentration also accelerates the aging of the red blood cell. Because about 95% of the oxygen transported in the blood occurs in combination with the hemoglobin inside red blood cells, these changes represent a generalized loss of oxygen supply throughout the body. However, like so many of the detrimental changes produced by blood sugar elevation, improved glucose control enhances the oxygen-carrying capacity. For diabetic athletes, one result of good glucose control is improved endurance. Conversely, poor control reduces endurance.

The immune system, including the white blood cells that fight infection, does not work at optimal levels when blood sugar is elevated. When combined with reduced oxygen being provided from the blood and damaged blood vessels, it is no wonder that many diabetics experience a reduced healing rate from infections.

In short, many physiological functions appear to be affected by the abnormal state of prolonged elevation of blood sugar levels. Physical growth and pregnancy are also affected, and the list could probably go on and on. However, awareness that these problems do so often occur in diabetics at least makes us recognize the importance of good diabetic control. The objective of good control should now be clear: maintenance of normal blood sugar as frequently and for as long as possible. You will probably experience fewer of the problems described and you will also function far more effectively in everyday living if your blood sugar is well regulated.

Existence of these problems in so many diabetics is a sad story. Diabetes is too often characterized as an "opathy problem," in reference to neuropathy, nephropathy, retinopathy, or diseased nerves, kidneys, and eyes, respectively. However, we can exert a high level of control of our blood sugar *if* we adopt a lifestyle that could serve as a model for everyone with some important particulars added. Furthermore, consistent long-term maintenance of normal blood glucose may partially, and in some cases totally, reverse many of the medical problems previously mentioned. So, although the health data on diabetics do not portray a very rosy picture, bear in mind that the data are skewed by many diabetic people not in good control. Blood sugar assessment at home was not feasible until recently; it wasn't realized until recently that many damaging effects of diabetes may be reversible. Lastly, perhaps not enough people with diabetes have truly lived a lifestyle in which blood sugar was adequately controlled. Today one might view the picture differently. If enough of us make use of today's technology and information, the health profile of the diabetic population, including *yours*, could be drastically changed.

chapter 2

Good News for Diabetics

As previously mentioned, many of the health problems to which diabetics are prone are related to elevated blood sugar levels. Consequently, it is not surprising that these conditions can often be reversed when blood sugar is better controlled. What's more, research in medicine has provided more precise information about how blood sugar can be better regulated. Technological development allows us to measure glucose levels daily in the comfort and convenience of our own homes rather than only periodically at the doctor's office. The means for better control are available and people with either type 1 or type 2 diabetes today can possibly prevent or at least delay damage to the eyes, kidneys, nerves, and blood vessels.

The benefits of good diabetic management (that is, good control of blood sugar via appropriate insulin or medication, diet, exercise, and glucose assessment) are many. Good diabetic management reduces the risk of diabetic complications to the eyes, nerves, blood vessels, and kidneys. Damage to these organs and tissues is highly related to the degree of blood sugar elevation. The frequent and prolonged rise in blood sugar damages the microscopic capillaries supplying blood to these structures, which deprives them of adequate oxygen.

Exercise and Diabetic Management

Endurance exercise, a basic component of the overall diabetic management program, reduces cholesterol (total cholesterol and LDL-VLDL cholesterol). Cholesterol is carried in combination with protein in a molecule called a lipoprotein (lipo referring to lipid or fat). Lipoproteins are categorized on the basis of the size and density of the fatty molecule component into three types: high, low, and very low density, or HDL, LDL, and VLDL, respectively. The first type of cholesterol, the HDL, is inversely related to heart and vessel disease, meaning that the higher its level the less frequently heart and blood vessel problems occur. The opposite, however, is true for the LDL and VLDL types of cholesterol. As a higher percentage of cholesterol is carried in these forms, more heart and vessel disease is observed. Aerobic exercise elevates HDL cholesterol, and reduces LDL and VLDL cholesterol and triglyceride. Adequate exercise also reduces a number of other cardiovascular disease risk factors. As body fat is reduced, blood pressure tends to drop, the tendency for the blood to clot is reduced, uric acid level in the blood drops (elevated uric acid tends to crystallize in the joints to produce gout), and stress can be reduced as well as tolerated more effectively.

Every time the blood sugar rises much beyond the normal range, the blood fat level rises and becomes the main energy source for most tissues in the body. It is this frequent elevation in blood fat that is believed to cause the greater than normal risk of cardiovascular disease in diabetics. Maintenance of blood glucose in the normal range will directly affect the amount of fat in your blood and therefore, your risk of cardiovascular disease. When exercise is used as part of the overall diabetes management program it often enhances the ability to maintain good blood sugar control. Exercise burns up glucose and glycogen within the skeletal muscles. During and after exercise, glucose from the blood enters the muscle (if the diabetic is well regulated) to build the glucose and glycogen levels back to normal levels. Whereas a sedentary diabetic's blood sugar may rise too high after a meal or snack, the physically active diabetic has a larger margin for error because if too much glucose is in the blood, some of it will be taken up by the exercised muscle mass. This reduces the tendency for hyperglycemia to occur.

Endurance training may reduce the likelihood of severe insulin reaction because it allows trained muscles and the liver to store more glycogen. During exercise it takes longer for muscle and liver glycogen to be used up. If the muscles become glycogen depleted and the blood sugar drops, the liver is stimulated to release glucose into the blood. In a trained individual the liver contains more emergency glycogen. Furthermore, trained muscle uses more fat and less glucose/glycogen during exercise, which reduces the breakdown of muscle and liver glycogen.

Good diabetic management will reduce the tendency toward ketosis. Ketosis promotes the breakdown of protein while good glucose control saves protein for more normal use (e.g., maintenance of muscle mass, white blood cells, enzymes, and hormones). Ketosis also increases red blood cell destruction, which reduces the capacity of the blood to carry oxygen, increases white blood cell destruction, which decreases the function of the immune system to prevent or recover from colds and infections, and increases the loss of electrolytes (minerals such as sodium, potassium, calcium, and magnesium) in the urine. The loss of electrolytes makes the heart prone to arrhythmia (abnormal heart rhythm), reduces muscle strength, and causes muscle cramps.

Weight Loss and Control

A program of sound diabetic management helps type 2 diabetics lose weight. The vast majority of people with diabetes are type 2 (about 85% to 90%) and about 75% of these people are overweight. Exercise of the proper type and amount can be very effective in reducing body fat, adding muscle, and improving physique. Because the loss of weight in type 2 diabetes, along with exercise, reduces the amount of oral medication needed, exercise is of particularly great value to persons with this type of diabetes. One chapter has been devoted to weight control because of its importance to those with type 2 diabetes.

People with type 1 diabetes are typically lean or of average body fatness. It has been my experience that many of us with type 1 diabetes often wish to add a few pounds. Good blood sugar control helps the process because when the blood sugar is elevated, protein and fat are broken down in larger than normal quantities to provide energy for the body. By reducing the extent of protein and fat breakdown, body weight can be added. Many people with type 1 diabetes note that body weight actually increases over several days of large amounts of exercise. More protein is synthesized, more sugar is stored in the muscles (more glycogen), which increases bulk and weight because water is stored with the glycogen, and the breakdown of muscle protein is minimized.

Muscular Fitness

Appropriate exercise will enhance your muscular fitness. You will become stronger, have improved local muscle endurance, and greater power (power = strength × speed or the speed with which work can be done). Endurance activity will improve your aerobic or cardiorespiratory endurance. You will be able to transport more oxygen in your blood, your heart will be stronger, and consequently will pump more blood per stroke or contraction (stroke volume). This will allow your heart to beat more slowly at rest and during submaximal exercise and to pump more blood each minute during maximal exercise. Endurance exercise will also increase the oxidative capacity of your muscle tissue. Your exercised muscles will develop more and larger mitochondria (the structure in cells where oxidation occurs), and have more enzymes (enzymes speed up chemical reactions). During exercise, the presence of more oxidative enzymes speeds the liberation of energy from the oxidation of carbohydrate and fat. The muscles will also be better supplied with blood. These changes will allow you to work and exercise longer and more vigorously.

Stretching will enhance your joint flexibility. With regular exercise the range of motion through which your limbs can move will improve. This enhances performance in sports and even daily activities such as turning backward to look behind you while driving a car. Good flexibility can minimize injury if you fall and it allows you to move more efficiently and comfortably.

Reduced Need for Medication or Insulin

With improved blood sugar control and consistent exercise, some people with type 2 diabetes can possibly eliminate the need for blood sugar-controlling medication. Both a reduction of body fat and increased physical activity enhance the function of insulin receptors lining the cells. Insulin receptors are chemicals that lie on the outside of cells to enhance the passage of glucose into the cell. With more receptor sites and/or better functioning sites, less insulin or medication is needed to allow normal metabolism in the cells. Adult-onset (type 2) diabetics typically produce a normal or even larger quantity of insulin than nondiabetics, but their insulin receptors do not work effectively. As most of the oral medications have some side effects, reduction or elimination of medications that assist in glucose control is beneficial.

Physical activity increases the function of the insulin receptors, which reduces insulin requirement. Endurance-type exercises also burn a considerable number of calories during the activity and the body continues to burn calories at an elevated rate for several hours afterward. In the first several months of an endurance-type exercise program, diabetics typically reduce their daily insulin by about 20% to 40%. Conversely, extremely sedentary living in nondiabetics increases their secretion of insulin in order to maintain normal blood sugar. This phenomenon has also been observed in American astronauts after several days of prolonged inactivity during weightless flight. It's no wonder that today's astronauts exercise during flight.

Improved Self-Image

A number of studies have demonstrated that physically active people feel better about themselves. They have improved self-images and self-concepts. Because much of what we actually do in life is in part a reflection of how we feel, it seems logical that a reasonably lean, physically fit diabetic who takes charge of his or her condition will accomplish more in life. Furthermore, although the research on the relationship between blood glucose and emotions is sparse, maintenance of normal blood sugar has always seemed to me to be a key determinant of how I feel emotionally. Most of us with diabetes have probably experienced the irritability and loss of emotional control associated with extremely high and low blood sugar levels. But notice how good you tend to feel while in the normal range. This "feeling good" phenomenon alone is reason enough to attempt to achieve normal sugar levels.

Coping With Stress

I have often noted that my tolerance to stress is powerfully affected by my blood sugar. Stress is a part of life and the controlled diabetic is less likely to overreact to it. Furthermore, exercise is an effective means of coping with stress. A pituitary gland secretion called beta endorphin is known to be secreted in larger quantities during exercise. Its effects include pain reduction and achievement of a relaxed psychological state. It has also been theorized as a possible explanation of "runner's high" or the perception of great energy and sense of inner tranquility reported by many joggers.

In summary, there are a number of persuasive reasons why those of us with diabetes should make all efforts possible to keep our blood sugar controlled. The benefits include avoiding or delaying many medical problems and, perhaps as important, simply feeling better emotionally. These possibilities would seem to fully justify doing all in your power to maintain proper blood sugar levels through a balance of exercise, diet, insulin or oral medication, and blood sugar testing.

Table 1   Benefits of Good Blood Sugar Control with Appropriate Exercise, Diet, Insulin, and Blood Sugar Assessment

1.   Reduced problems with eyes, nerves, blood vessels and kidneys
2.   Reduction of cardiovascular disease risk factors
3.   Enhanced ability to maintain good blood sugar control
4.   Reduced tendency toward ketosis
5.   Improved physical fitness and sports performance
6.   Reduction and possible elimination of medication to control blood sugar for noninsulin-dependent diabetics
7.   Reduced insulin requirements for insulin-dependent diabetics
8.   Improved self-image and self-concept
9.   Greater tolerance of stress

chapter 3

Components of Good Diabetic Control

This chapter deals with the regulation of blood sugar, which is the basis for achieving good diabetic control. You will better understand the fundamentals of good diabetic control by realizing the differences between the two types of diabetes. The characteristics of type 1 (insulin-dependent) and type 2 (noninsulin-dependent) diabetes are summarized in Table 2.

Three major factors regulate blood glucose in diabetes: insulin or oral blood sugar-lowering medication, diet, and physical activity. The sum of the effects of each factor determines blood sugar level. The interaction of the factors is represented in Figure 1. Note that each factor exerts an effect on blood sugar. For example, exercise will lower blood sugar if there is adequate insulin in the blood. Eating obviously will raise the blood sugar while insulin or oral medication will reduce it. Blood sugar measurement therefore provides an index to the overall balance of the three factors. Maintenance of blood sugar at desirable levels is somewhat complex because of the number of factors affecting it and because of the inconsistencies of daily living. For example, your caloric expenditure may be considerably lower during weekdays as compared to weekends if you work in the yard or if you pursue other physically active hobbies on the weekends. We have to

Table 2 Characteristics of Type 1 and Type 2 Diabetes

Characteristics	Type 1 or insulin-dependent	Type 2 or noninsulin-dependent
Former terminology	Juvenile-onset	Adult-onset
Age at onset	Usually before 20	Usually after 40
Family history	Infrequent	Frequent
Appearance of symptoms	Rapid	Slow
Use of insulin	Always	Common but not always required
Production of insulin by pancreas	Absent or greatly reduced	Usually normal or elevated
Proneness to ketoacidosis	Prone	Not prone; rarely occurs
Body fatness	Usually normal or lean	Often obese

make allowance for these differences. Although diabetics typically control diet by consuming food on a measured basis, differences exist in how the body handles different types of food. Diet for diabetic individuals is consequently more complex than the mere counting of calories or food exchanges. For example, a half cup of orange juice will elevate the blood sugar faster than will a slice of bread although both are equivalent in calories. A serving of oatmeal will tend to release its energy more slowly than a serving of cornflakes, as will an apple compared to a glass of apple juice. However, the response of the blood sugar (that is, how fast and how high it rises) to eating a specific food varies from person to person. Diabetic individuals need to identify foods that cause an overly rapid rise in blood sugar and eat those foods selectively.

Stress typically elevates the blood sugar via the release of the adrenal hormones. (However, in some type 1 diabetics, stress can reduce the blood sugar.) The impact can be quite

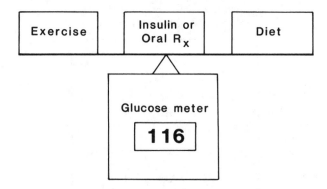

Figure 1   Regulation of blood sugar through the interaction of exercise, insulin or oral medication, and diet

significant in emotionally charged situations. For example, several hours prior to an athletic event, nervousness and anxiety may cause the blood sugar to rise. If this rise occurs at approximately the same time as a scheduled snack, eating the snack may cause an elevation in blood sugar high enough to detract from performance.

The purpose of these examples is to demonstrate the day-to-day variability in physical activity, stress, and diet. For diabetics, these variations may pose problems unless care is taken to account for the effect of these variations. The obvious answer is to measure your blood sugar at regular intervals during the day as well as during times of unusual circumstances such as athletic events, travel, illness, holidays, and in times of stress. Knowledge of your blood glucose at such times allows modification of insulin, diet, or exercise to bring you back to a level of control. Without this precise information, you have little or no potential for making appropriate adjustments.

The remainder of this chapter deals with guidelines that can be used to maintain good diabetic control (or good blood sugar control). Figure 2 schematically summarizes the use of blood sugar testing in a sound diabetic management program.

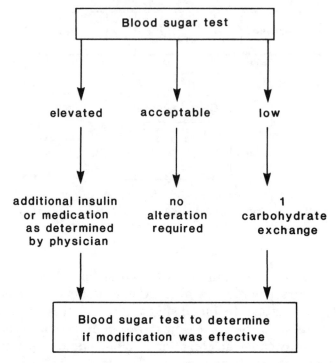

Figure 2   The use of blood sugar testing in the management of diabetes

Blood Sugar Assessment

Accurate measurement of blood sugar is the critical first step you can take to achieve good diabetic control. The only truly accurate means of doing this is to measure the sugar in the blood directly. Urinalysis is very prone to error as it reflects the content of sugar in the blood in the hours urine is being formed. For example, your blood sugar may be 160 mg% (or 160 milligrams in one-tenth of a quart or liter of blood [100 dl or deciliters]) 1 hour after lunch, and some of this excess sugar (normal = 70 to 110 mg%) will likely spill into the urine. However, if one didn't urinate in several hours, urinary sugar could well show positive and possibly mislead you into thinking you should take extra regular insulin to reduce the sugar level or eat less at the next feeding. Either action may lead to low blood sugar and insulin reaction. Urinalysis in this example may be misleading and cause you to begin treatment for high blood sugar when the blood sugar may actually be normal or even low at the time. A second disadvantage of urinalysis is that the blood sugar level at which excess sugar spills into the urine (called the renal threshold for glucose) varies from one person to another. In many people with diabetes this occurs at about 130 to 160 mg% but the variation can be quite large. People with high renal thresholds may consequently get negative urinalyses, while the blood sugar level at that time may actually be fairly high.

Prior to the availability of blood glucose monitoring kits for home use, diabetics were cautioned to perform urinalysis only after a second voiding or urination about 30 minutes or so after the first. In theory, this works well as a second urine sample would contain extra sugar only if it appeared in the blood during that 30-minute interval. However, my experience and discussion with diabetics in the days when urinalysis was used indicates it was hard enough to get them to do a urinalysis at regular intervals much less to do one after a first voiding. Undoubtedly, this second voiding situation also presents a problem simply because of limited time. If you urinate soon after arising, by the time you are able to void a second time you may already be driving to work or may be at work, and by that time you probably have eaten breakfast. Consequently, urinalysis done only on the first voiding in the morning does not represent your actual blood sugar at that time; hence no corrective action can be taken if it is high or low. Because of these limitations I "hung up" my Tes-Tape several years ago.

The major advantage of having your own blood sugar measuring instrument is accuracy. All the limitations of urinalysis are eliminated with today's devices. The instruments are easy to use and maintain and require only poking (I like this word better than "puncturing"; the latter sounds like an injury) a fingertip to obtain one good-sized drop of blood. "Hold it!" you say. "I already have to stick myself once, twice or thrice daily with a needle." However, I will vouch for the ease and minimal discomfort produced. Most of us who have been doing this for a while don't bat an eyelash at the procedure. It is no more painful than our injections and besides, we get to do the sticking. When you're the one in control, perhaps psychologically you don't mind it as much. Furthermore, by using the side of the fingertip where fewer nerve endings are located, the discomfort is reduced. Devices are now commercially available that automatically do the procedure. A spring-loaded lancet contained in a pen-like device makes the process simple and nearly painless. Also, I find it comforting to know I am using the best of modern technology. The cost of electronic blood sugar kits has recently dropped considerably in the last several years. Formerly costing over $300, they can now be purchased for about $150 and it is quite likely that your physician can write a letter to your insurance carrier recommending that you purchase it. My insurance company picked up the whole bill and I believe that has become fairly typical.

You can purchase chemical strip indicators to use without the electronic measuring device. The same procedure is used; that is, the fingertip is punctured and a drop of blood is placed on the strip of chemically coated material at one end. After waiting for a designated time and rinsing or wiping the end of the strip, its color is then compared to a chart on the container. Each color represents a specific blood glucose value. However, I've never felt confident in my ability to interpolate or make a measurement where the color seems to be between two values. Too frequently you wind up having to estimate. While this is still considerably better than urinalysis, it is not as precise as the digital or numerical readout where numbers appear on a viewer on the electronic models.

So, the directly measured blood sugar analysis is infinitely more accurate, the purchase will most likely be refunded by your insurance carrier, and it is fast and easy to perform. I view it as a necessary piece of equipment for those of us with type 1 diabetes. If you have type 2 diabetes, its value will be proportional to the degree that your blood sugar tends to fluctuate.

The target glucose levels recommended by diabetologists that diabetics should attempt to attain are 60 to 130 mg% before meals, 140 to 180 mg% 1 hour after meals, and 120 to 150 mg% 2 hours after meals.

Consistency

As previously stated, life doesn't seem to allow perfect consistency. Each day of our lives is different with many factors influencing our blood sugar. Consequently, alterations must be made in insulin, diet and/or exercise. However, those of us with diabetes will do well to keep certain facets of our lives as constant as possible. That implies waking up and retiring at the same time each day, administering the same amount of insulin at the same time(s), and eating and exercising at the same time. By doing so, you can simply determine the best combination of variables to use in regulating your blood sugar. Then, when exceptions to your lifestyle do arise or can even be anticipated, adjustment is facilitated. For example, if blood sugar tends to be high or low for several days at about the same time of day, it is markedly easier to alter one aspect of insulin/diet/exercise that is a relative constant in your day. In this case, you might adjust either insulin or food to correct the problem. It has been my observation that a factor related to the principle of consistency is that good blood sugar control appears to facilitate continued blood sugar control and conversely, loss of control seems to inhibit ensuing control. In other words, a balanced state seems to promote a balanced state.

Multiple Daily Insulin Injections

Recent evidence indicates that normal blood sugar levels in type 1 diabetics can realistically be accomplished all or most of the time only if insulin is administered continuously or numerous times throughout the day, including prior to any feeding. This observation is noteworthy because it points out the limitation of the single injection. It is also interesting to note that multiple injections mimic the release of insulin in the nondiabetic's normal functioning pancreas. The explanation for this centers on the length of time in which a given insulin provides a blood sugar-lowering effect and the time required for this effect to begin once administered. Table 3 summarizes this information for the most frequently used types of insulin. Rapid-acting insulin such as regular begins its effect about 1 or 2 hours after being injected and lasts approximately 6 hours. Intermediate-acting insulins such as lente and NPH begin their effect about 6 hours after administration, and the effect is sustained for about 24 hours. Because of these factors, a once-a-day dosage of only intermediate-type insulin would not facilitate the movement of glucose into the cells after breakfast. Therefore, such a regimen would tend to promote high blood sugar (hyperglycemia) in the middle and late morning. To prevent such an occurrence, diabetics (insulin-dependent) typically use a mixture of insulins such as regular and intermediate. The regular insulin would take effect an hour or two after breakfast depending on how soon before breakfast it was injected. Diabetics prone to midmorn-

Table 3   Speed and Duration of Glucose-Lowering Effect of Various Types of Insulin

Type	Time until peak effect (hrs.)	Duration of effect (hrs.)
Regular	2	6
Semilente	3	12
NPH, lente	6	24
Protamine zinc	16	36
Ultralente	20	36+

ing sugar elevation might be advised to take their insulin a good 45 minutes or so prior to breakfast to receive the effect of the regular insulin that much sooner after breakfast. Figure 3 illustrates the insulin pattern presently used by the author.

The overall goal of this pattern is to provide some blood sugar-lowering effect throughout the day and night. I take extra regular insulin before breakfast, dinner, and an evening snack to control the surge of glucose entering the blood following these feedings. I don't require regular insulin before lunch because I usually exercise soon afterward. I use lente insulin (intermediate) in the morning and at 5 p.m. to provide for a long-lasting control of my blood sugar during the day and night. When two types of insulin are mixed and injected simultaneously, this is called a mixed-dosage regimen. Most diabetics who take insulin more than once a day administer about two thirds of the day's total before breakfast. However,

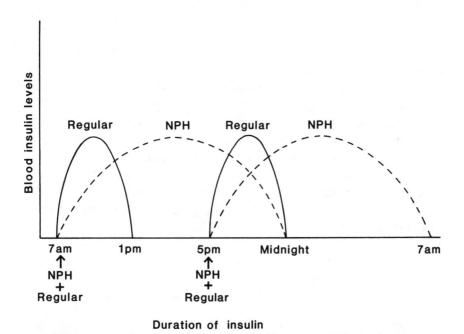

Figure 3 Blood insulin levels over 24 hours using a multiple injection, mixed-dosage regimen (Regular + NPH)

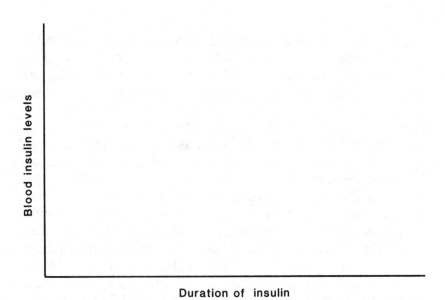

Figure 4 Graph of when your insulin(s) has its peak blood sugar-lowering effect

every diabetic's regimen will be somewhat different depending on his or her needs.

Plotting the activity of your insulin(s) over 24 hours is a valuable means of determining when you will have the tendency for both low and high blood sugar. Use the graph in Figure 4 to sketch in your own insulin-glucose curve(s). It should be realized also that the sketch can be useful in knowing when and how to make modifications in insulin, diet or exercise. The important concept to understand is that the timing of meals and exercise should be related to the timing of the peak effect of your insulin(s).

Correction Plan

If you have type 1 or type 2 diabetes, what can you do when your blood sugar is elevated? Should a meal be skipped or reduced in calories? Should extra insulin be taken? Should you take extra medication? These questions have to be answered by diabetics, particularly those with type 1, more frequently than they care to admit. Therefore, it is helpful to have a structured, carefully planned procedure established. Your physician or nurse-educator probably provided you with such a plan when you were first diagnosed as diabetic, but the plan needs periodic modification based on changes in your life such as growth, physical activity, and stress. A "correction plan" should include the following:

1. A plan for low blood sugar
    It is recommended that just one carbohydrate exchange in a rapidly digestible form such as orange juice or candy be used for treatment of insulin reactions. Although low blood sugar can greatly increase the appetite, you must resist overeating and causing a rise in blood sugar. However, if symptoms of low blood sugar are not relieved within 20 minutes, an additional carbohydrate exchange should be taken. Beyond this, I would take additional food only if warranted by a blood sugar test below about 70 mg%. Do not let your appetite govern how much you eat as you will typically overeat.

2. A plan for high blood sugar
    a. Some physicians recommend that their patients take extra regular insulin to lower blood sugar to a normal range whenever it exceeds a certain level. I use 150 mg% for my threshold. However, those with type 2 diabetes are not as prone as type 1 diabetics to dramatic rises in blood sugar. Because insulin is produced in type 2 diabetics, taking additional insulin could result in a precipitous fall in blood sugar. For this reason, those with type 2 diabetes should discuss a correction plan to treat high blood sugar with their physicians.
    b. If you have been advised by your physician to take regular insulin when your blood sugar is elevated markedly, how much regular insulin should you take? One unit of regular insulin will typically lower the

blood sugar about 40 to 50 mg% if the blood glucose is in the range of 150 to 200 mg%. As the sugar rises, more insulin is required to lower the sugar level. Therefore, if we consider normal as 100, then a reading of 200 would warrant taking 2 units of regular insulin; 260 may require 3 or 4 units, and so on. If your glucose rises to 300 mg% or higher, you should check your urine for ketones. If you are ketotic, your physician will probably suggest a dosage of regular insulin. The blood sugar and urine ketone level will have to be carefully monitored. If the sugar and ketone levels do not begin to drop, you may have to be hospitalized to prevent severe ketosis and possible coma. Ketosis is a life-threatening condition and you should contact your physician if it occurs.

I do not recommend taking more than 4 units of "corrective" insulin unless your physician recommends it, as it represents a potent blood sugar-reducing force several hours later. Larger amounts of insulin also require a longer time to exert their effect than smaller amounts. A follow-up blood glucose test is warranted when you have taken supplementary insulin as a corrective measure to assess whether or not the sugar has reached the normal range. Until the follow-up test you should be on guard for possible insulin reaction. I would also urge caution regarding exercise in this period as it may accelerate the absorption of insulin into the blood and hence speed up the lowering of blood sugar. Also, never exercise if you are ketotic because this will increase ketone production and cause a further rise in blood sugar. A snack normally taken in this period should be delayed until the follow-up blood sugar test to determine if it is actually needed.

part II

Physical Fitness

chapter 4

Special Concerns for Exercising Diabetics

Exercise has many beneficial effects for diabetics and non-diabetics alike. When performed at least three times weekly, it will enhance blood sugar balance and total diabetic well-being. One can readily understand, therefore, why regular physical activity is a vital component in the diabetic program.

My training as an exercise physiologist has been very helpful in making adjustments in my insulin, diet, and exercise pattern. The effects of exercise on biochemistry are rather complex but I have found a number of facts useful in allowing exercise to be very helpful in controlling blood sugar. All too often I have heard people with diabetes speak of problems with insulin reaction during or following exercise, so this chapter includes tips based on applied physiology that can help you prevent such problems.

Energy Cost of Various Activities

It is helpful to know the approximate number of calories expended in physical activity and the extent to which it will affect the blood sugar. Table 4 provides data about the number of calories expended in a wide variety of sport and daily activities. These data are more accurate than others because they consider the effect of body weight. Notice that body weight needs to be considered because it has a large effect in determining the energy or calorie cost of most activities. The accuracy of the data is somewhat limited, however. The values represent averages and make no account for individual variations. For example, one could play volleyball or half-court basketball with many varying levels of intensity and consequently varied levels of energy expenditure. The table is most accurate for activities in which the speed or intensity is relatively constant such as walking, jogging, cycling, and swimming. However, in group activity, the pace and energy expenditure are strongly influenced by skill and the level of competition.

In diabetics exercise lowers the blood sugar only if a functional amount of insulin is in the blood. If the blood sugar level

Table 4   Estimated Calories Expended Each Minute in Common Work, Conditioning, and Recreational Activities[1]

Activity	Weight in pounds				
	100	130	160	190	220
Work Activities					
Mowing lawn	3.8	4.9	6.0	7.2	8.3
Chopping wood	4.9	6.4	7.9	9.3	10.8
Shoveling	5.3	6.9	8.5	10.1	11.7
Digging	5.7	7.4	9.1	10.8	12.5
Conditioning Activities					
Level walking					
One mile in:					
30 minutes	1.9	2.5	3.0	3.6	4.2
24 minutes	2.6	3.4	4.2	5.0	5.8
20 minutes	3.4	4.4	5.5	6.5	7.5
17 minutes	4.2	5.4	6.7	7.9	9.2
15 minutes	4.9	6.4	7.9	9.3	10.8
Level jogging					
One mile in:					
12 minutes	5.7	7.4	9.1	10.8	12.5
10 minutes	6.3	8.2	10.0	11.9	13.8

(Cont.)

Table 4 (Cont.)

Activity	Weight in pounds				
	100	130	160	190	220
8 minutes	6.8	8.9	10.9	13.0	15.0
7 minutes	9.1	11.8	14.5	17.3	20.0
6 minutes	11.4	14.8	18.2	21.6	25.0
5 minutes	15.0	19.5	24.0	28.5	33.0
Level Bicycling					
One mile in:					
11 minutes	2.3	3.0	3.6	4.3	5.0
10 minutes	2.6	3.4	4.2	5.0	5.8
6.5 minutes	3.8	4.9	6.0	7.2	8.3
4.5 minutes	6.8	8.9	10.9	13.0	15.0
Swimming: crawl stroke					
1 ft/sec	3.8	4.9	6.0	7.2	8.3
2 ft/sec	7.6	9.9	12.1	14.4	16.7
2.5 ft/sec	11.4	14.8	18.2	21.6	25.0
3 ft/sec	20.0	19.5	24.0	28.5	33.0
Calisthenics	3.4	4.4	5.5	6.5	7.5
Sports and Recreational Activities					
Canoeing, 2.5 mph	1.9	2.5	3.0	3.6	4.2
Horseback riding, walk	1.9	2.5	3.0	3.6	4.2
Volleyball, 6-people recreational	2.3	3.0	3.6	4.3	5.0
Bowling	2.6	3.4	4.2	5.0	5.8
Horseshoes	2.6	3.4	4.2	5.0	5.8
Golf	3.0	4.0	4.9	5.8	6.7
Ballroom dancing	3.4	4.4	5.5	6.5	7.5
Table tennis	3.4	4.4	5.5	6.5	7.5
Tennis	4.5	5.9	7.3	8.6	10.0
Horseback riding, trot	4.9	6.4	7.9	9.3	10.8
Folk dancing	4.9	6.4	7.9	9.3	10.8
Skiing	6.0	7.9	9.7	11.5	13.3
Horseback riding, gallop	6.0	7.9	9.7	11.5	13.3
Squash	6.4	8.4	10.3	12.3	14.2
Fencing	6.8	8.9	10.9	13.0	15.0
Basketball	6.8	8.9	10.9	13.0	15.0
Football	6.8	8.9	10.9	13.0	15.0
Handball	7.6	9.9	12.1	14.4	16.7

[1]Adapted from Wilmore, J.H. (1986). *Sensible fitness*. Champaign, IL: Leisure Press.

is elevated to about 300 mg% or higher, exercise will usually increase the blood sugar. Furthermore, if ketones are present in the blood, exercise will result in even greater production of ketones. Therefore, use of the data in Table 4 for diabetics is only valid if your blood sugar is under control.

It is useful to estimate the number of calories expended in your typical exercise session because it helps to understand why insulin requirement may drop markedly in the first several months of an exercise program. Secondly, it provides a better understanding as to why exercise has a potent effect on weight and body fatness. One pound of fat yields approximately 3500 calories. If you expended 300 calories each day in exercise and exercised 5 days weekly, the weekly energy cost equals 1500 calories. At this rate, 3500 calories (or 1 pound of fat) would be expended in 2.33 weeks. This figure may not be impressive, but if the effect is carried out over 6 or 12 months, then the impact seems considerable. In 6 months, you would lose 11.2 pounds and in a year the loss would be more than 22 pounds! That is particularly impressive when it is realized that no dietary restriction is included in the figures. Also, the data in Table 4 do not include the calories burned during recovery. When you complete an exercise session, your metabolism or energy expenditure remains considerably elevated for several hours. This is particularly so when exercise is vigorous and prolonged. For example, running a marathon costs approximately 3000 calories (depending on body weight, speed, and efficiency) and the metabolism remains elevated for more than 24 hours. With more typical 20- to 30- minute sessions, the increased energy in recovery may last several hours. So, the total energy cost of physical activity exceeds that listed in Table 4.

Energy Sources During Exercise

While at rest, the tissues of the body utilize a mixture of fat, carbohydrate, and protein to provide energy. The role of protein is typically rather small, about 3% to 5% of the total energy. The contribution of protein does not change even during strenuous exercise until exercise duration exceeds about 2 to 4 hours. For individuals with diabetes, however, at about 40 minutes into exercise protein metabolism provides a higher percentage of the total energy supply. Fat and carbohydrate are still the major sources of energy.

The proportion of energy supplied by fat and carbohydrate, however, does vary considerably depending on the type of exercise. In short, intense types of exercise such as weight training, sprinting, and any exercise performed all-out for several minutes, carbohydrate (i.e., glucose and glycogen) provides nearly all of the energy. In light to moderate work where the oxygen consumed each minute is less than 50% of maximum, fat is the major energy supplier. This would include activities like walking, cutting grass, and gardening.

A second factor in this energy relationship is the duration of the exercise session, which to a degree is dependent on the intensity. For example, realistically one can't sprint for more than about 20 to 30 seconds. The longer the duration of an exercise, the lower its intensity must be. As one exercises for longer periods, carbohydrate becomes progressively less used as an energy source while fat becomes a relatively more important source. For example, consider a fit person running at about 75% of his or her maximum for 45 minutes. In the first 20 to 30 minutes, carbohydrate is the major energy supplier with fat as the secondary source. As one exercises longer than about 30 minutes, fats become the major source of muscle fuel with carbohydrate as a secondary source. As exercise duration becomes longer, fat becomes an increasingly important fuel. With exceedingly long activities such as backpacking and recreational cycling where the oxygen consumed is typically about 25% to 50% of maximum, fat provides about 60% to 75% of all the energy. Figure 5 illustrates these relationships. Understanding the extent that fat and carbohydrate are used as muscle fuels during exercise is important because it means that our blood sugar is not equally affected by all types of exercise. Again, it should be noted that the exact degree that fat and carbohydrate provide energy can only be determined individually. The shape of the curve is affected

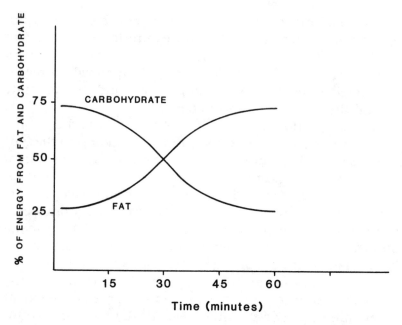

Figure 5   The effect of exercise duration on the proportion of energy supplied by carbohydrate and fat during exercise at 75% of maximum effort

by exercise intensity such that if you ran all-out in a 10 kilometer road race (6.2 miles) in 45 minutes, the contribution of carbohydrate would be significantly higher than if you jogged the same distance considerably slower. Also, as musculature becomes better conditioned over many weeks of endurance-type exercise, the muscles begin to use more fat and less carbohydrate for energy. Thus, a trained diabetic is less likely to deplete all the muscle carbohydrate (glycogen) during exercise and so is less likely to have to depend on the relatively small amounts of glucose/glycogen in the blood and liver. The net result of training thus allows one to exercise longer before being prone to low blood sugar and depleted muscle glycogen. In addition, endurance training causes the trained muscles and liver to store extra glycogen; this too inhibits "running out of sugar."

Diabetics typically utilize fat for energy during exercise more extensively than nondiabetics. This may be a result of having less glycogen stored in our muscles due to periods where we don't have adequate insulin in our blood.

The Effect of Exercise on Insulin Requirement

As previously noted, when adequate insulin is present in the blood, exercise enhances the absorption of glucose from the blood into muscle tissue. Chronic exercise also increases the sensitivity of the insulin receptors lining the cells of muscle, liver, and other tissues. This results in less insulin or medication being needed to move a given quantity of glucose out of the blood and into the tissues. In adult-onset or type 2 diabetes, regular exercise can sometimes allow total elimination of insulin or oral medication used to assist in blood sugar control. This particularly seems to be true when substantial weight is lost and the diet includes a high proportion of complex carbohydrates. In insulin-dependent diabetics, insulin will still be required regardless of activity level but the quantity is typically decreased by about 20% to 40%. That's a very dramatic change and should be considered by any diabetic initiating an exercise program. One study demonstrated that 20 to 30 minutes of jogging 5 days weekly dropped insulin dosage by 30% to 40% while another study noted a 75% reduction during several days of backpacking!

How can you determine how much to decrease your insulin when beginning an exercise program? I know of no formula or way to predict the extent of insulin reduction as it would vary with the length and intensity of exercise, whether or not it was done daily, the amount of body fat present, the fitness of the person, and so on. Again, the best feedback will be the results of your blood sugar tests. In the early weeks of an exercise program I recommend doing several extra blood sugar assessments daily, recording the results, and then making adjustments in insulin with the advice of your doctor. Just knowing what to expect and the general change you will be making (that is, a decrease in insulin) should be helpful. Realize too that as you get in better condition, your muscles will use fat as an energy source to a greater extent and consequently a continued drop in insulin requirement will slacken and at some point will eventually cease. Also, remember that exercise will only decrease the blood sugar if you are taking adequate insulin. Exercise will increase the blood sugar if it is high (about 300 mg% or higher) at the start.

Planning Ahead for Exercise

To minimize problems with insulin reactions, type 1 and type 2 diabetics should consider "all the angles" or variables. First, relate the time of day you will be doing the exercise to your insulin-glucose curve (discussed in Chapter 3) by answering the following questions:

1. Will your insulin(s) or medication be exerting its peak blood sugar-lowering effect at the time of exercise?
2. How long will it have been since your last meal or snack?

Answers to the above questions will help you decide if you need to eat a snack prior to exercising. I generally prefer exercising during the noon hour on weekdays and in the mornings on weekends. On weekdays, I eat a light lunch such as a piece of fruit and a sandwich about an hour before my exercise. Research indicates that in healthy people, a light meal low in fat and less than 500 calories does not impair physical performance. I'll vouch for that as I have comfortably done my exercise in such a manner for nearly 30 years. The intervening hour allows time for my stomach to settle and by the end of the hour I am probably getting a gentle rise in my blood sugar. That's a good time for diabetics to begin an exercise session.

A rule of thumb that has stood the test of time for me has been to check my blood sugar prior to exercise anytime I feel irritable or nervous. These symptoms may mean either low or high blood sugar. If my sugar is low, I eat additional food (one carbohydrate exchange) and delay exercising until I feel better. If my sugar is high, I take a supplemental dosage of insulin only if above about 200 mg%. Combining insulin with exercise accelerates the drop in blood sugar because exercise accelerates the absorption of insulin into the blood.

One has to be cautious in doing this. In such an instance I closely maintain a vigil for symptoms of low blood sugar. It should also be emphasized that if you have been out of metabolic control and ketones are present in the urine, then exercise should be avoided because exercise while ketotic makes the condition even worse. Let me emphasize this point as on several occasions years ago I didn't realize this. I thought exercising while hyperglycemic and ketotic would lower my blood sugar. During these exercise sessions I probably felt the worst I have ever felt while exercising and on each occasion I suffered for several hours afterward until additional regular insulin straightened me out. So, if ketones are present, blood sugar control should be reestablished before exercising.

Type 2 diabetics can also experience an insulin reaction during or after exercise, so they too should be alert for symptoms. It would be wise to inform your doctor of your intention to begin an exercise program. Your doctor will probably reinforce your decision to start a program but he or she can also give you specific guidelines about reducing your medication.

The Effects of Insulin on the Capacity to Exercise

Insulin facilitates the movement of glucose into the tissues and decreases the production and release of glucose by the liver, thereby having a blood sugar-lowering effect. When excess insulin is present in the blood, however, it also inhibits the breakdown and utilization of fat as an energy source. This leads to an exaggerated use of glucose/glycogen by the muscle tissue and an even faster potential drop in blood sugar. So, if one administers extra insulin as a corrective measure and then also plans on exercising, the likelihood of insulin reaction can be high. It also should make you wary of exercising while your insulin may be exerting its peak effect, unless you eat a snack first. Because of this effect, it is interesting to note that a study of diabetic long-distance runners reported that the majority of them reduced or eliminated the quantity of regular insulin in their morning dosage on days when competition occurred in the morning. These runners also purposely attempted to have their blood sugars mildly elevated immediately prior to exercise. It should also be appreciated that these runners were competing in races of more than 6 miles to as long as 26.2 miles.

Injection Site

Injection of insulin into a region of the body that will shortly be active in exercise accelerates the absorption of insulin in the blood. Consequently, the time to peak insulin effect and decreasing blood sugar is shorter. For this reason, if one plans on running, cycling, or skiing in the early morning, the thigh may not be a suitable injection site as each of these modes of exercise extensively involve the quadriceps muscles of the frontal thigh. If lifting weights or swimming soon after injection, the arm or shoulder would not be an appropriate injection site. The abdomen and gluteal regions do not seemingly alter the speed of insulin absorption and so may be effective sites in such cases. It has been speculated that these areas are not affected much by exercise because of the relatively thick layer of fat present. Fat is not abundantly supplied with blood vessels that may slow the absorption of insulin.

I also use this knowledge to more rapidly lower my sugar when attempting to self-correct a high sugar reading. I do notice that injection into the shoulder or arm followed by three sets of push-ups does speed my return to normal.

The Day After Extensive Exercise

An experience common to physically active diabetics is having low blood sugar problems the day after a day of unusually high levels of physical activity. For example, years ago when I was first getting into long distance running I had two mild insulin reactions the day following my first half-marathon race (13.1 miles). At that time, that was considerably farther than my longest training run and so I was unprepared to handle the resulting drops in blood sugar. Exercise of long duration such as distance running, backpacking, hiking, and even yard work expends considerable energy. You can enjoy a bit larger snack and meal to compensate on such occasions. This will allow you to meet the energy needs during the period of activity. However, I was often surprised that I needed to continue eating more the next day as well. The reason for this is that muscle tissue has a limited store of glycogen, which is the storage form of glucose. Although fat as well as carbohydrate (glycogen) are used for energy in long periods of physical activity, the continual burning of glycogen can nearly totally deplete the muscle and the liver of glycogen. Many of the calories needed the following day are used to refill the muscle and liver with glycogen. So, you should be prepared for needing extra food. I even carry an extra supply of hard candy on such days, as low blood sugar often has occurred in periods of the day where I normally don't tend to have problems, such as midmorning.

Summary

1. If initiating an exercise program, be prepared to reduce your overall insulin or oral medication requirement.

2. Estimate the number of calories you will expend per session. Increase or decrease your intake of food to match the extent that the exercise will deviate from the normal amount.

3. Try to exercise at about the same time of day to facilitate planning.

4. Plot the time of peak blood sugar-lowering effect of each of your types of insulin. If planning to exercise at about the same time, plan to take a light snack 20 to 30 minutes prior to exercise.

5. Do not exercise if ketones are present in your urine or if blood sugar is above 300 mg%.

6. If you feel "funny," irritable, or nervous prior to exercise, check your blood sugar.

7. If planning an unusually large amount of physical activity, be prepared to eat additional food or to reduce your insulin. If choosing the former, light snacking every 30 to 60 minutes will help ward off insulin reactions. Be prepared for low blood sugar the following day; carry extra candy in your pocket or purse.

8. Alter the site of your insulin injection if subsequent exercise would allow the insulin level in the blood to rise too quickly. Avoid the arms and shoulders if planning to do weight training or swimming; avoid the thighs if running, cycling, playing basketball, or doing aerobic dance. Speed of absorption of insulin from the abdomen and gluteal area seems to be minimally affected by exercise and may be a suitable alternative site in such instances.

chapter 5

Principles of Exercise

Over the last several decades, researchers in physical education and medicine have established a number of principles that optimize the safety and efficiency of exercise. The principles apply to males and females of all ages.

Consult Your Physician

Prior to starting a fitness program, consider if you should consult with your physician. If you have diabetes, talking to your doctor is particularly important because exercise affects blood sugar. A number of details should be discussed with your physician including the amount of insulin or medication taken, when the exercise should preferentially be done, and whether a snack prior to exercise is needed. The other factor to be concerned with is your health status. If you have been a smoker, have elevated cholesterol, or if heart disease has occurred in your family medical history, your doctor may want to assess the function of your cardiovascular system with a graded exercise treadmill test. The test not only serves a diagnostic function, that is, identification of any defects in the heart or blood vessels, but also allows you and your physician to determine an appropriate starting point for your exercise program.

The importance of the medical checkup cannot be over-emphasized. We have all read of veteran joggers who may have reached the point of believing they are completely resistant to disease, particularly cardiovascular disease, because they have run a number of marathons and because for several years they have logged a huge quantity of running miles. Jim Fixx, the author of the running book that was on the best-selling list several years ago, comes to mind. He had been overweight and a smoker for a number of years prior to becoming a jogger. His years of jogging may have improved his health and fitness greatly, but the disease process in his arteries may have occurred in the less active days when he was a smoker, or he may have had a disorder in his body's ability to handle fats, which was not altered by his exercise regimen. On either account, he ignored symptoms of angina pectoris, which is the sensation of pain and pressure in the chest and left shoulder, and even rejected an offer for a free treadmill test at the Aerobics Research Institute in Dallas. So, regardless of your age, fitness level, or how you feel, let your doctor pass judgment on what diagnostic tests are needed and how you can safely begin an exercise program.

A number of universities offer sophisticated fitness testing and counseling services including treadmill testing, underwater weighing to determine body fatness, and assessment of muscular fitness with an electronic instrument called a Cybex dynamometer, which measures muscle force and endurance of selected joints. Contact the physical education department at a college or university, and if they have an exercise physiology or human performance laboratory, chances are you can make use of their expertise for a reasonable fee.

Start Comfortably

Start your exercise program at a comfortable level and progress slowly. Common sense suggests beginning an exercise program easily and progressing on a gradual basis. However, if there is one common fault I have observed people making in initiating a fitness program, it is failure to adhere to this principle. I think the problem stems from impatience. People have visions of the desired end-product and can't wait to get there. So, many jump right into a regimen that would be more appropriate for them after 6 months of gradual progression. The consequence is undue soreness and stiffness, which does much to dampen their motivation. If your first experiences are painful, the probability of continuing the activity is significantly diminished.

I have seen far too many runners in the early months of conditioning come down with a rash of orthopedic overuse injuries. We test and counsel many such individuals in the Exercise Physiology Laboratory at the University of Nebraska at Omaha, which I direct. They are typically well motivated but have simply gone at it too quickly; they have done too much exercise too soon. It is frustrating to them when an orthopedist or exercise physiologist tells them they must either slow down, stop the activity, or switch to a different activity. If an injured runner has to stop running for 6 weeks to allow an injury to heal, he or she loses some of the conditioning for running. So, the result of rushing into things too quickly is a delay in progress. Figure 6 illustrates the progress attainable under a crash program leading to periodic injury versus that of a program characterized by small increments in progression. The comparison is analogous to the race between the hare and the tortoise: The overall progress is usually greater in the person who trains conservatively because injury is avoided. A second benefit is that avoidance of injury allows you to reap the psychological benefits and pure enjoyment of exercise on a more consistent basis. Because consistency of lifestyle enhances blood sugar control, avoiding injury perhaps takes on increased importance for the diabetic.

The physiology of injury is not only interesting but a brief explanation of it may motivate you to progress gradually. The rate that various tissues adapt to a conditioning stimulus appears to vary. Endurance capacity increases fairly quickly; that is, heart and skeletal muscle adapt quickly. However, response of the connective tissues (such as bone, cartilage, tendon, and ligament) is a bit slower. The result is that after

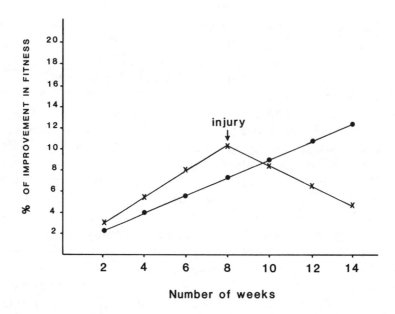

Figure 6   Comparison of improvement in a "crash" program versus a program where progression is gradual

a month or two of endurance exercise, you typically have the
staying power to dance, jog, cycle, or swim at a moderate pace
for a prolonged time; but for the connective tissues, the time
may be excessive. This may be true particularly when exercise is done daily. Connective tissue is apparently slightly
damaged as a result of vigorous exercise. That is not as bad
as it sounds, because the damage is temporary and is followed
by a period of physiological adjustment in which the tissue
is strengthened in a process called supercompensation. The
critical factor as related to injury of the connective tissue is
the relationship between the extent of damage and the extent
of repair or supercompensation. If there is a consistent mismatch in favor of damage over a month or two, then at some
point injury will occur. Bending a coat hanger once produces
little noticeable damage, but as the stress-induced damage
continues, the effect soon becomes significant. The key then
is to allow adequate time for compensation and to closely control the extent of damage done. A useful tip regarding the latter
is to use muscle soreness as a guideline. Recent research in-

dicates that muscle soreness only occurs when connective tissue has been damaged. So, whenever one has exercised to the point that pain is experienced, further exercise of the same type probably makes it difficult for the rate of connective tissue repair to catch up with the extent of damage. In such a case, one is probably better off to use a different form of exercise. For example, sore runners could use swimming or cycling as a substitute; weight trainers with sore arms or shoulders could do aerobic exercises using the legs, and so on.

Warm-Up and Cool-Down

Warm up before every exercise session and cool down afterwards. Warm-up is more than a mere formality. Its purpose is to (a) increase the temperature of muscles, which increases both the velocity as well as the force of the contraction, (b) heat connective tissue making it more elastic, thereby decreasing the chance of pulls or tears as well as increasing the efficiency of joint motion, (c) speed chemical reactions within muscle cells, which provide energy for muscle contraction, and (d) increase the flow of blood and with it, oxygen, to the muscle cell. The net effect of warm-up is to enhance strength, speed, power, local muscle endurance, flexibility, efficiency, and cardiorespiratory function.

The value of warm-up as a safety factor should not be minimized. When one begins exercise without warm-up, muscle tissue is not provided with enough blood and oxygen to allow most of the energy to be produced through oxidation. Therefore, some energy in the first several minutes must be produced without oxygen or anaerobically, which results in the production of the waste product lactic acid. These chemical changes (that is, increased acidity, low oxygen, increased lactic acid) decrease the efficiency of the contracting muscle. What is experienced in the first several minutes of exercise without warm-up is a fatiguing of the muscles, an associated physical discomfort, labored breathing, and an overly high heart rate. If one has a heart condition, this rapid rise to a level of heightened physiological overload can lead to chest pain or angina pectoris, dangerous changes in heart rhythm, and possibly even a coronary. So, heart patients or anyone even with heart disease risk factors should make sure to warm up appropriately.

It is recommended that warm-up last a minimum of five to ten minutes and consist of light exercise. Joggers/runners would do well to walk a distance, then stop and do some calisthenics and stretching, and then finally begin jogging at a speed well below that which makes one huff and puff. The sequence of light activity followed by calisthenics and easy stretching followed in turn by gradually increasing work effort until one reaches the target heart rate level is a safe, effective procedure that is even used by Olympic and professional athletes. You will certainly feel better as well as perform more effectively after having warmed up thoroughly.

Notice that I have relegated the role of stretching in the warm-up process to one of secondary importance. This was done intentionally. Stretching, by itself, does not accomplish any of the aforementioned objectives of warm-up. Secondly, stretching relatively cool connective tissue seems to be illogical as it probably is not as easily elongated when cool, and forced stretching may actually tear it. So, if you feel bound by tradition to stretch prior to the stimulus or conditioning part of the workout, at least do it after 5 to 10 minutes of whole body light exercise when the connective tissues are heated. Or, stretch at the end of the cool-down when you know the tissues are considerably warmer and more pliable.

The mild exercise done after the main portion of a workout is called cool-down. It consists of low-intensity exercise followed by stretching. One purpose of cool-down is to provide an adequate flow of blood to the muscles to enhance the removal of lactic acid. We always form some lactic acid in muscles even when the work intensity is not particularly high. If you don't remove some of the lactic acid, muscle stiffness and soreness seem to be greater the day or two following the exercise session. So, cool-down facilitates lactic acid removal and thereby reduces muscle discomfort.

A second reason for cool-down is to enhance the return of blood in the veins to the heart. Every time we walk a step or move a limb, muscles in the extremities contract and squeeze the veins, "milking" the blood back to the heart. Without cool-down, if a person suddenly stood still or sat down immediately after exercise, the heart would be deprived of enough blood to the extent that the amount of blood it pumps suddenly would decrease. Consequently, blood flow to many tissues would suddenly decrease, resulting in dizziness, headache, seeing spots in the field of vision, and nausea. To avoid these potential unpleasant side effects, keep moving for 5 to 10 minutes after exercise, and then stretch the muscles at the end of the cool-down.

Consistency

To obtain a significant training effect and maintain it, one must exercise at least two or three times a week. However, once a reasonable level of fitness is attained, two sessions each week maintain a surprisingly good portion of the gains made.

Because diabetics achieve a better sugar balance when each day's energy expenditure is relatively constant, I think it is best to be physically active in some form nearly every day. This may sound extreme, but I think as one goes through several months of exercise, it tends to become a very enjoyable part of each day. It can provide a chance to "blow off some steam," socialize, and relax. My almost daily runs in certain seasons give me the opportunity to be alone, which at times is what my psyche seems to need. Being off alone with nature and hearing your breathing coupled in pace with your footsteps has a soothing, calming effect. Whether or not "runner's high" is caused by hormonal changes is controversial, but I am fully convinced that many people would benefit psychologically from occasional periods of being alone. Exercise can provide the opportunity.

Total Fitness

Several different types of exercise are needed for total fitness. Physical fitness is comprised of aerobic fitness, muscular fitness, flexibility, and body fatness, and each type of fitness requires a specific type of training. Consequently, runners who only run may lack muscular fitness in the arms and shoulders, as well as flexibility. To be totally fit, you need to stretch and perform aerobic exercise as well as strength-type exercise. Aerobic exercise not only builds aerobic fitness but also is effective in decreasing body fat because it allows a substantial expenditure of energy.

Progression

The exercise stimulus must be progressive in order to improve fitness. If I lifted a 75-pound barbell 10 times every Monday, Wednesday, and Friday for the next 6 months, little improvement in strength or muscle endurance would be demonstrated after the first week or so. So it goes with aerobic fitness and flexibility. If you bicycle at the same speed and for the same time several days each week, your aerobic fitness reaches a plateau. That's not to say plateauing is bad; if you have raised your strength or aerobic fitness to a level with which you are satisfied, there's nothing wrong with sustaining it. For most people, this is a realistic approach to physical fitness. Only competitive athletes need to be concerned with trying to attain greater performance levels by forever increasing the exercise stimulus. But, when you wish to raise your fitness level, progression must be made. One must either do more total work or work more intensely.

chapter 6

Aerobic Fitness

Experts in health, medicine, and fitness believe that aerobic fitness is the single most important component of physical fitness because of the numerous health benefits it provides, including the reduction of heart disease risk factors. While it may appear that these benefits are of value primarily to adults, studies regarding the health status and physical activity of children indicate otherwise. In our laboratory we tested a sample of elementary school children and found that 42% of the children had at least one coronary heart disease risk factor. Based on national health statistics 8% to 13% of the children were considered to be at risk for each of the following risk factors: high blood pressure, elevated cholesterol, excess body fatness, and low aerobic fitness. Other researchers have found similar results. Another study monitored the amount of intensity of physical activity in children by having them wear portable EKG units for several days. They observed that only 13 minutes per day were spent in vigorous activity (i.e., greater than 160 beats per minute) and this figure represented an accumulated time rather than a continuous time. The purpose in describing these data is to emphasize that children may not be as physically active or as fit as one might suspect. Children spend considerable time sitting behind a school desk and in nonschool hours they may spend quite a bit of time watching television, using a computer, or playing video games. Therefore, the fitness requirements of children may need to be more structured or planned than previously thought. For diabetic children, this may be helpful not only from a fitness standpoint but also from the basis of blood sugar control. Furthermore, encouraging vigorous daily physical activity in children may establish a habit and expectation of fitness that may transfer to their adult years. Just as diabetic children must learn how to administer their own insulin and test their own blood sugar, they should also realize the importance of physical activity in the control of their condition and learn to partake of some activity on a daily basis.

Aerobic fitness is important for people of all ages, but to elicit an aerobic conditioning effect in children or adults, four factors should be considered: intensity, duration, frequency, and mode. Simply said, unless you exercise hard enough, long enough, and frequently enough, and select aerobic activities, you will not improve your aerobic fitness. The threshold for each of these factors will be described in this chapter.

Intensity

To obtain an aerobic training effect, exercise or work must be vigorous enough to reach at least 50% of a person's maximum ability to use oxygen in producing energy. This capacity is expressed as the amount of oxygen used per kilogram (2.2 pounds) of body weight per minute. Direct measurement of this maximum oxygen consumption capacity or max O_2 uptake is done in a laboratory setting where a person walks and jogs on a treadmill or rides a stationary cycle. Figure 7 shows the equipment used in the author's exercise physiology laboratory for this test. The initial workload is very low and every several minutes the workload is increased in small increments. During each workload or stage, a mouthpiece is used to direct expired air through tubing into instruments that measure the volume of air expired each minute as well as the percentage of the expired air that is oxygen and carbon dioxide. A computer is usually interfaced with these instruments to calculate the amount of oxygen consumed by the person each

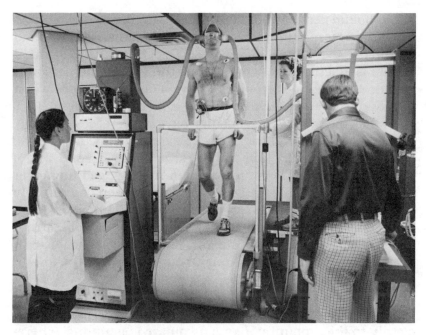

Figure 7   Equipment used to measure maximum oxygen uptake
on a treadmill

minute. So, as each stage of the test is performed, the computer feeds information such as the oxygen consumed to a printer, which types the data. As the workload progressively rises so does the quantity of oxygen consumed. The largest quantity of oxygen consumed usually occurs in the last minute of exercise when you are working at maximum capacity. During the test, your ECG or electrocardiogram, heart rate, and blood pressure are monitored to indicate if your cardiovascular system is functioning properly. If a symptom such as chest pain occurs during the test, the test is immediately stopped. Thus, the test is an excellent diagnostic tool to assess the health of the heart and blood vessels, but it also indicates the relative state of endurance capacity of the muscles used in walking, running, or cycling, depending on whether the test was performed on a treadmill or cycle.

The max O_2 uptake score is expressed relative to your body weight so that people of varying weights can be compared.

A 220-pound person would be expected to consume more oxygen in the last minute of maximum exercise than a 120-pound person due to the great difference in size. But if the 220-pound person is inactive and overfat while the 120-pound person is lean and active, the latter may have a far better score when the total oxygen is divided by his or her body weight.

While the capacity to consume oxygen decreases with age, the scores of physically active people clearly indicate that the reduction of this function can be rather small. In one study, the max O_2 uptake was measured in middle-aged men over a 10-year span. While the scores of inactive men consistently decreased a bit each year, the highly active men showed no change in their capacity. Other studies have indicated that the decrement in maximum oxygen uptake each year in vigorously active people is only about one half of the loss in sedentary people.

The heart rate during exercise can be used as an index of how vigorously you are exercising because it is related very closely to the amount of oxygen you are consuming. Therefore, if you exert to a level where your heart rate (HR) reaches 60% of maximum, this is roughly equivalent to 50% of the max O_2 uptake, which is also the threshold in untrained people for obtaining a training effect. The question that logically arises is, what is the best intensity, as measured by a percentage of the maximum heart rate, for each person? The maximum heart rate gradually declines with age, and in people for whom the HR max is not directly determined during a treadmill test, it can be estimated by subtracting their ages from 220. For example, a typical HR max for a 20-year-old is about 200 (220 − 20 = 200); for a 40-year-old it is about 180 (220 − 40 = 180). Realize, however, that this procedure is but an estimate. Some 20-year-olds may have a HR max of only 190 while others may be well over 200 beats per minute.

Next, one needs to determine the percentage of this directly measured or estimated HR max that is appropriate for your health and fitness status. I recommend starting at 60% of HR max if you are sedentary, have a fitness level below average, have been or presently are a smoker, or if you have any medical limitations such as a heart-lung disorder. As previously stated, any adult beginning a fitness program should consult with his or her physician before starting. Any diabetic should also receive guidance from a physician regarding how to develop an exercise program.

Most young, healthy individuals with diabetes can comfortably begin at about 70% of maximum HR, and for those who have been quite active in endurance-type activities, 80% to 90% would be appropriate. Little or no extra health benefits come from exerting beyond this point. Most people would find it quite tiring and uncomfortable to exercise beyond this intensity because quite a bit of the energy produced within the muscle would be through nonoxidative processes leading to a rise in muscle and blood lactic acid. This acid inhibits muscle contractility, which leads to fatigue. Consequently, most people find high intensity exercise very uncomfortable and they are unable and/or unwilling to sustain the exercise long enough to obtain a training effect.

A different formula to estimate the target or exercise heart rate is:

resting HR + 60% to 90% (max HR − resting HR)

The former procedure as well as the one above both require knowledge of the max HR. Because HR max decreases fairly steadily with age, it should be understood that the final calculation of the target HR will be considerably lower in older persons. For the elderly, the target HR may be as low as 110 to 120 beats per minute, while in adults aged 20 to 40 the threshold typically ranges from 130 to 150 beats per minute. As indicated previously, selection of a value between 60% to 90% is based on one's health and fitness level. The same criteria explained previously can be used in identifying the proper value in this formula.

To obtain a valid measure of the resting HR, do so at a time when you are emotionally calm because emotions exert a great effect on heart rate. Also, take the measure several hours after having eaten and consumed caffeine or nicotine as these factors also elevate the heart rate. Remember that many soft drinks as well as tea, cocoa, and chocolate contain caffeine.

A useful guide that indicates if you are accumulating lactic acid in the muscle while exercising is the presence of labored breathing. When you begin to huff and puff it signals lactic acid buildup. The rise in this acid and other byproducts of exercise metabolism are carried by the blood to the portion of the brain that regulates breathing. As the acidity of the blood rises, the frequency and volume of breathing increase. This phenomenon occurs at about 55% to 60% of the max O_2 capacity in untrained college-aged people and ranges as high as 85% to 90% in elite endurance athletes. In very sedentary people, it often is about 30% to 40% of maximum. Regardless of your age or fitness level, huffing and puffing indicate that you should slow down and recover for several minutes before returning to a more comfortable pace.

While monitoring the heart rate during exercise is useful in terms of exerting at an appropriate intensity, I don't feel you must depend solely on it and I don't believe it must be taken numerous times during an exercise session. Interrupting movement to monitor heart rate detracts from the flow and continuity of movement, and the enjoyment. The only exception is for people with defined exercise limitations such as cardiovascular disease. If you take the pulse rate three or four times each session (about every 5 minutes) this will provide a frequent enough check. After several weeks of activity, you will likely find you can quite accurately gauge the appropriate exercise intensity without frequent HR monitoring by "listening to your body," that is, attending to feedback regarding your breathing, body temperature, and general sense of fatigue. At this point, taking your pulse rate twice each workout will provide an adequate check for most people. Veteran exercisers typically do not measure their heart rates during exercise.

Measuring pulse rate or heart rate is a simple procedure that requires just a bit of practice to master. By placing moderate pressure with two or three fingers over any large superficial artery, you can feel the alternating expansion and reduction in the size of the artery as blood passes through. As the heart contracts and squeezes blood into the large arteries, blood flow is momentarily increased, which distends the walls of the arteries. As the heart relaxes blood flow is reduced, which allows the artery to recoil to its resting diameter. This alternating change in size allows us to measure how rapidly the heart is beating. Consequently, measurement of pulse rate is an indirect measure of heart rate.

Several sites are commonly used to measure pulse rate. One is the carotid artery, which lies just beside the voicebox. It should be noted that a small percentage of people can become dizzy or faint when putting pressure on this artery, so if this should happen, choose a different site. A second location is the radial artery located on the thumb side of the wrist. Place moderate pressure at one of these sites and you should be able to feel the pulse. If you have difficulty, try a number of sites and realize that if you apply too much pressure, you may block the flow of blood through the artery, thereby making it impossible to feel the pulse. A third location is the chest wall directly over the heart. Because the heart is a fairly large organ, about the size of the fist, placement anywhere over it allows one to readily feel the heart beating. This is particularly so during exercise because the heart contracts more vigorously during exercise and ejects about 50% more blood per stroke or contraction as compared to rest; therefore, it's easier to feel.

It is important to take the pulse rate as soon as possible after you have stopped moving. Once you stop, the rate rapidly decreases. If it takes you 5 to 10 seconds to locate the pulse and another 10 seconds to count, the pulse may have slowed 20 or more beats per minute. Therefore, the pulse rate you take would be significantly lower than it actually was while you were exercising. Practice will allow you to begin taking your pulse almost immediately after stopping, and if you take the pulse for only 6 seconds, the reduction in pulse rate should be quite small. Use of the 6-second pulse count also simplifies the computation to convert the pulse count to beats per minute: You only have to add a zero. For example, 13 beats in 6 seconds is a heart rate of 130 beats per minute. If you count the pulse rate for 10 seconds, multiply by 6 to obtain the rate per minute; a 15 second count is multiplied by 4. These are not exactly complex mathematics, but I have seen even college students stand for a few moments performing the mental calculation or even scrawling the numbers on dirt. Counting longer than 15 seconds after exercise will result in a significant error.

Duration

The minimum time required for aerobic conditioning is about 15 to 20 minutes per session at target heart rate level. However, longer sessions will accelerate progress, burn more calories, and contribute to greater reduction in the serum lipids (cholesterol and triglyceride). However, orthopedic injuries increase significantly when people go to longer sessions particularly if they involve running or jumping. Most beginners would be wise to limit each session to 15 to 20 minutes in the first month or two in order to minimize overuse injuries. From there you can gradually progress to 30-minute sessions because this duration provides several advantages (e.g., greater weight loss and reduction in blood fats). Exercise beyond this time represents a point of diminishing returns in terms of the overall conditioning response. Because warm-up and cooldown should each last at least 5 minutes, the minimum time for each aerobic exercise session is 25 minutes (5 minutes for warm-up, 15 minutes at the target rate level, and 5 minutes for cool-down).

Frequency

At least two or three training sessions are required each week. People with very low fitness levels can initially make improvement with only two weekly sessions, but after a month or two, they will then require three or more sessions to make further progress. Three sessions per week will maintain aerobic fitness for most people but not for the highly trained. For people with diabetes, I think daily exercise is advantageous because it makes energy expenditure more constant, facilitating maintenance of good blood sugar control. The exercise on other days can be less vigorous and less structured since the goal on these days need not be actual conditioning but more for blood sugar control and, for noninsulin-dependent diabetics, for weight control as well.

Mode

Any physical activity that uses many large muscles for a sustained period and elevates the heart rate to a threshold level will provide aerobic conditioning. This description implies use of the legs and includes activities such as jogging, brisk walking, backpacking, swimming, cross-country skiing, rope jumping, aerobic dance, soccer, basketball, racquetball, and bicycling.

Because approximately half or perhaps even more of the aerobic training effect occurs in the muscles that are used during exercise, if one uses several types or modes of exercise, then the conditioning effect of any one muscle group is reduced. For example, in cycling, the frontal thigh muscles are used more extensively than in running, which uses the posterior thigh muscles or hamstrings more extensively. So if a person jogged 2 days each week and cycled 2 other days, the frontal thigh muscles as well as the posterior thigh muscles would be lesser trained than if one had done all four sessions using just one of the two activities. In terms of energy expenditure, serum cholesterol and triglyceride, and other health-related benefits of exercise, this training effect is not important. Many people enjoy a variety in exercise, which in turn makes it easier for them to maintain their exercise programs. In my own exercise program, I like to include several differ-

Table 5 Summary of Criteria for Aerobic Conditioning

Fitness/training level	Intensity (% max HR)	Frequency (days/week)	Duration (minutes)
Low, beginner over age 35, medical limitation	60%	2-3	15-20
Intermediate, average, adolescent & young adult	70-80%	3-5	30
Advanced, motivated, competitor	80-90%	4-7	30+

ent activities. Jogging and bicycling are my favorites in good weather, but I sure enjoy some occasional soccer and basketball in the driveway. From a physical performance standpoint, however, one is provided a better effect by primarily using one activity. For example, a competitive runner will demonstrate a greater gain in performance by running nearly every day rather than cycling 2 days weekly, swimming 2 days weekly and running only 3 days weekly.

A summary of the criteria for aerobic conditioning appears in Table 5.

Other Considerations

The maximum oxygen uptake and the gains made in maximum O_2 uptake as a result of training appear to be strongly affected by heredity. Top level athletes in endurance-prominent events such as middle- and long-distance running and cross-country skiing usually have maximum O_2 uptakes exceeding 70 units per minute (that is, 70 milliliters of O_2 per kilogram of body weight each minute) and often well into the 80s, whereas average college-age males score about 45 to 50 and college-age females score 35 to 40. With training, typical gains in max O_2 uptake are about 5% to 30%. A 5% and 30% improvement for a person with an initial score of 50 units of oxygen would raise the max O_2 uptake to 52.5 and 65 units, respectively. However, a 30% increase is generally limited to those who are initially unfit and overweight. More realistically, achievement of a score much above 60 units may indicate some level of genetic endowment. It is also interesting to note that a gifted athlete even in a state of relative detraining will generally score higher than many moderately trained people with little or no hereditary advantage. An example is Jim Ryun, former world record holder for the mile. At his peak, his max O_2 uptake was 81 units of oxygen. A year after retiring from competition in which he did little training, his score dropped to 65, which for Jim represented a tremendous drop in fitness. However, many of us who have trained for years will never approach 65 units. Even when I was running more than 50 miles weekly for over several months training for a marathon, my score was only 55 units.

Selection of Appropriate Physical Activities

As previously mentioned, if one has been sedentary or is obese, jarring activities such as jogging, rope jumping and aerobic dance should be avoided. Selection of appropriate activities should focus on doing things that you will enjoy, won't hurt you, and can be done individually. Realization that any exercise using many large muscle groups is equally effective should encourage people to select activities they enjoy. While some, like myself, really like jogging and running, it's pure boredom for others. The activities we choose may in part be a reflection of our personalities. Some have proposed that people with an ectomorphic or long, linear bone structure tend to be introversive and consequently select activities that can be done alone and in a state of relative peace and quiet. People with heavier, more rugged physiques supposedly crave more exciting activity as well as socialization, and therefore select activities that can be done with others. Running would seemingly appeal to the ectomorphic group while tennis, racquetball, and aerobic dance done in a group would be preferred by the more outgoing people. The theory is interesting but scientifically unsubstantiated. It is mentioned here only to offer it for whatever value it may have in helping you to select appropriate activity.

In trying to think of different activities, be practical. If you are overweight and don't want to exercise in public or at least in skimpy exercise clothing in public, exercise at home with a stationary cycle or rebounder. If limited time is a problem in trying to start an exercise program, then spending time driving across town to a YMCA or other facility may prove frustrating.

Progression

Fitness gains will occur only if the training stimulus is increased. One has a choice of exercising longer, harder or more days per week. Whatever the choice, to minimize overuse injury, progress in small increments. For example, sedentary adults might consider the walking regimen in Table 6. The progression here is based on increasing the duration but it increases only 5 minutes every 2 weeks. This may seem very conservative but if aches, pains, injuries, and doctors' bills are to be avoided or minimized, in the long run it is the best

Table 6   Starter Walking Program for Sedentary Adults[1]

Week	Duration (minutes)
1 and 2	15
3 and 4	20
5 and 6	25
7 and 8	30
9 and 10	35
11 and 12	40

[1]Intensity or walking speed which elicits 60% of maximum HR

way to proceed. In the initial 12 weeks I also advise previously sedentary people to walk only three times each week on alternate days. When and if a person has completed the 12th week without any discomfort, then further progression may be accomplished by increasing the frequency of exercise or the intensity. For example, one might walk 4 or 5 days each week or remain at 3 days each week but walk at 65% of maximum heart rate rather than 60%.

Increasing the intensity of exercise is advantageous because it allows a greater conditioning effect without increasing the time spent in exercise. However, when the intensity reaches a certain level, the connective tissues are stressed more, inviting injury. Furthermore, at a certain level of strain, the activity is not as enjoyable or relaxing. Because of these factors, my advice is to seek an intensity of exercise that maintains your fitness and body weight at a desirable level and yet doesn't require an inordinate amount of time. In other words, seek the combination of these factors that fits your lifestyle, mood, and available time. And again, for those of us with diabetes, I strongly believe that daily exercise of some sort aids in keeping our blood sugar level more constant. This doesn't necessarily mean that a daily workout where the HR is monitored is required, but it may include household chores such as cutting the grass, gardening, snow shoveling, or playing catch.

Let me remind you, too, that exercise does not have to be overly intense to provide an adequate training effect. One study demonstrated that in a group of university professors, walking four times weekly for 40 minutes produced equivalent gains as a jogging program consisting of three sessions weekly for 20 minutes. Look at exercise as a potentially enjoyable way to stay healthy. Search for activities that will be enjoyable enough that you will look forward to an exercise session of some sort each day.

30 Minutes Daily

Aim eventually for at least 30 minutes of aerobic exercise three times weekly. On other days one could exercise for a few minutes less. The shorter sessions reduce the incidence of overuse injury but yet allow a reasonable number of calories to be burned and so favor a fairly constant insulin and eating pattern. Several advantages are associated with an exercise duration of about 30 minutes. One is that a significant number of calories are burned, which aids in weight loss and weight maintenance. Second, a significant change in the blood fats occurs: Total cholesterol, VLDL- and LDL-cholesterol, and triglycerides are all reduced while HDL-cholesterol is elevated. Remember that HDL-cholesterol is inversely related to cardiovascular disease (that is, people with higher levels of HDL are statistically less likely to have cardiovascular disease). It has also been my observation that exercise often doesn't tend to be really enjoyable until about 15 or 20 minutes into a session. This may in part be a reflection of the fact that this amount of time may be required for an optimal warm-up. Once thoroughly warmed-up, the muscles function better, the joints move more easily, and breathing becomes less noticeable. It's no wonder we feel good at this point because all systems are working optimally. Unfortunately, many exercisers stop at the time the body has reached this point and consequently miss much of the pleasure perceived during exercise. George Sheehan, a cardiologist, marathon runner, and leading philosopher and guru of the running movement, once stated that the first 30 minutes of running are for the body while the second 30 minutes are for the mind. He meant by this that 30 minutes of aerobic activity is adequate for the purpose of physical training, but that the most enjoyable and relaxing effects are experienced in the second half hour. I imagine that part of the explanation for this phenomenon includes the time it takes to relax. Today's rush-rush behavioral pattern leads us to react to many stimuli. When one gets off alone for a while running, walking, cycling, or swimming, stimuli such as the telephone, intercom, and colleagues' and clients' queries are left, and the alert, sometimes overaroused central nervous system can gradually unplug itself from the heightened workload. I often find that during the first portion of my daily run my mind is still very much back at the office contemplating the rest of the day's schedule, conversations I had with students or colleagues that morning, and so on. Gradually, these thoughts fade away and seem to be replaced by dominance of my sensory system. I become more conscious of my breathing, stride length and rate, and smoothness of my movements. The central nervous system appears to become relatively quiet and more reflective, perhaps because fewer high priority stimuli are arousing it. It's a pleasureful mode in which to operate.

Runners as a group frequently describe these feelings of tranquility, reflection, and pleasure while running. Some go as far as to term it a "high." Interestingly, some evidence suggests a possible link between the runner's high and the secretion of several hormones from the central nervous system such as norepinephrine and the beta endorphins. These chemicals seem to be released in greater quantities during exercise and their effects include mood elevation and pain reduction. So, there may be a biological basis for the runner's high. Runners who report these feelings typically indicate that the phenomenon does not occur until 30 minutes or more into an exercise session and only when the pace is moderate or easy.

Because stress is related to so many health problems, exercise duration several times weekly at or above 30 minutes may provide some of the previously described benefits, thereby reducing the impact of stress on one's health.

Environmental Effects

Many people like to walk or bicycle at about the same speed each day. For example, they may wish to walk each mile at a 20-minute mile pace. Although this may be a comfortable pace when the weather is fairly similar day after day, it may not be very comfortable if the weather is much warmer and more humid. Under such conditions, the physiological work load (e.g., heart rate) might be far higher than when walking the same speed on a cooler, dryer day. The heart rate would also increase, of course, when walking or bicycling uphill. If you were walking or cycling at a constant pace and then came to a hill, and if you maintained the same speed going up the hill, then more oxygen is needed, the heart has to beat faster and pump more blood, and so on. So if the goal is to maintain the heart rate at the target level when going uphill, then the speed has to be slowed somewhat. You can slow your pace to keep the effort fairly constant or you can expend more effort to keep the pace constant. The same would be true when walking, running, or bicycling into the wind or with the wind.

Another example of how one has to regulate exercise according to the environment is the effect of high altitude. The force of gravity is reduced as one goes away from the surface of the earth, and consequently, less oxygen is brought into the lungs per breath. This reduces the amount of oxygen carried in the blood. So if you are accustomed to a certain exercise pace back home where the elevation is 500 feet and you went to the mountains at altitudes exceeding 5000 feet, exercising at the same pace would produce a higher exercise heart rate. To exercise at the same HR as at home, you would have to slow the pace to match the relative lack of oxygen available to the tissues.

Energy Level

Each day requires a varying level of energy to cope with demands placed on us. Realization of this now allows me to accept blah-type days occasionally. Most days of my life I feel quite good and energetic, and once or twice a month I feel almost super. My blah days, on further analysis, can often be attributed to overly strenuous physical work on a preceding day, or to a cold or stress. I think I have learned to become less frustrated and concerned about not being able to exercise at the same pace each day. I simply don't attempt to do as much on such days. I usually slow the pace and run, bicycle, or ski a lesser distance. So don't fight it; let your energy level tell you what and how much to do.

Rope Jumping and Minirebounding

Many activities can be used to provide an aerobic conditioning effect. Research indicates that rope jumping and minirebounding may not necessarily provide the conditioning that one might expect. Rope jumping, for example, at a typical speed of 60 to 80 jumps per minute, is equivalent to the energy expended during slow jogging. Skipping rope at a high rate of speed much as a boxer or basketball player might at 120 to 140 times per minute raises the energy cost to a level that would be very similar to what the average recreational jogger expends per minute. For the athlete who is at a high level of fitness, even skipping rope at high speed may not provide an aerobic conditioning effect. Similarly, for those trying to develop a conditioning effect, slow jumping may not be intense enough. So, rope jumping, like any other activity, has to be gauged to meet the needs and capacity of the individual. Rope jumping, particularly in novices, involves considerable jarring and is probably not suitable for sedentary people initiating a fitness program. Any activity that involves jumping is very likely to produce muscle soreness and aches and pains. I generally recommend that people start off with nonjarring activities such as walking, biking, or swimming. Skilled rope skippers minimize the jarring effect by jumping no more than an inch or two off the ground; novices typically expend much more energy and magnify the impact at landing by jumping far too high.

Minirebounding has become very popular in the past 5 years or so in the United States, and while it is very appropriate exercise for some people, for relatively young and fit individuals, it probably will not increase the heart rate or oxygen consumption high enough to obtain a conditioning effect. We once tested a group of college students while they performed typical exercises on the device for 15 to 20 minutes. We found that they were not able to raise the heart rate to their target levels. However, for many older and less fit people, the minitrampoline or rebounder could be effective because it may provide the threshold of exercise that is appropriate for people with limited physical capacity. It also has the advantage of use in inclement weather and it minimizes the trauma to the joints and connective tissues.

Criteria for a Successful Exercise Session

Here is a simple way to determine if an exercise session was appropriate or whether it was too much, too strenuous, or too long. First, you should feel more refreshed, vitalized, alert and energetic after you have completed an exercise session. Secondly, exercise should make you feel good about yourself. If one meets frustration by failing to achieve unrealistic goals, then the psychological values of exercise are lost. The most relaxing and stress-reducing workouts are typically experienced by people in noncompetitive conditions. Life offers many challenges and if exercise becomes a means by which a person feels obligated to improve, it may raise anxiety and tension levels rather than reduce them. When this happens, you should consider if this tension is a positive or negative force in your life.

I enjoy occasional competition with others as well as myself, but I realize my limits. There are periods of the year when my work keeps me very busy and at such times, I've learned I cannot maintain the psychological and physical energy to train as hard as I might in the summer months. Learn to adapt your exercise regimen to the total demands placed on you, and you will be more likely to find exercise to be a balancing factor in your life rather than an additional stressor.

chapter 7

Muscular Fitness

Muscular fitness has two components: strength and local muscular endurance. Strength is the maximum force that you can produce in a single contraction, while muscular endurance is the ability to use your strength over a period of time. Strength is often measured by determining the heaviest weight that can be lifted one time. Muscle endurance is often evaluated by the number of pull-ups, dips, push-ups, sit-ups, and similar exercises that can be performed.

Importance of Muscular Fitness

Muscular fitness is considered a fitness component because it is related to the ability to perform work and sport effectively in our daily lives. While most people would not question the usefulness of strength and endurance in sport and recreational activity, it may be less obvious as to the importance of these factors in a typical day. However, strength and endurance partly determine posture and the susceptibility to a variety of joint problems such as lower backache, muscle tightness, and associated discomfort. Also, the ability to do yard work, assembly-line work, housework and other typical daily activities safely and efficiently is in part dependent on muscle fitness. Many injuries occur to people when changing a tire, painting, lifting objects, and gardening because the muscles and associated tendons lack strength. One medical authority has stated that the single most common cause of low backache is the lack of muscular fitness in the abdominal muscles. Strength training not only strengthens and enlarges the muscles but also increases the thickness and density of bone, and the strength and thickness of tendons, ligaments, and joint cartilage. Such changes in connective tissues occur as a result of the muscles pulling with substantial force on the bones to which they are connected. Progressive resistance training is probably the most effective way to promote these developmental changes. Consequently, a complete fitness program includes training to develop and then maintain a reasonable level of muscular fitness. As you will see, developing and maintaining a reasonable level of muscular fitness does not mean spending a lot of time or lifting stupendously heavy weights. Nonathletes, in fact, can get by very effectively with about 30 minutes per week using the weight of the body for resistance.

Training Principles

Following are descriptions of some training principles for achieving muscular fitness.

Exercise Through the Full Range of Motion

Researchers in physical education, physical therapy and physical medicine have determined that weight and resistance training will not decrease joint flexibility when properly performed. Often, flexibility will increase as a result of moving the limbs to the furthest positions in the beginning and end of joint movements. Many have observed the body builder or weight lifter who walks with his arms held far to the sides of the hips. This stance may result from the desire of the lifter to show off his muscle development and/or it may be the result of failing to straighten the arms completely at the beginning of each movement in rowing or curling type exercises. Connective tissue will shorten and create unnatural joint positions if one fails to completely straighten (extend) or bend (flex) the limbs in the beginning and end of most exercises.

Progressive Overload

A beginning weight trainer must initiate a program with rather light weights. This minimizes injury but also allows progress to be made readily, which enhances motivation. Correct performance of each exercise requires some learning, and working initially with moderate resistance facilitates this skill development. Bone growth in adolescents is not complete and lifting heavy weights may damage the region where bone growth occurs (called the epiphyseal plate). Damage to the growth center may interfere with the completion of bone growth. Working initially with light weights reduces the stress on the growth center and allows for a progressive strengthening of tendons, ligaments, bones, and cartilage.

As changes are made in the neuromuscular system, your strength will improve and a slightly heavier weight or resistance can be used. As long as you increase the resistance, then strength will continue to grow. The increments of weight added should be rather small to avoid strain and to allow completion of the appropriate number of repetitions of the movement without altering safe lifting technique.

Sets

A set is a unit of work in weight training. When a weight trainer lifts a barbell, performs a given number of movements, and then places the bar on the floor, one set has been completed. Research has indicated that performance of three sets of an exercise produces significantly greater levels of strength than doing either one or two sets. Performance of two sets, as a matter of fact, is not much better than performing one set.

I recommend in the early weeks of training that you perform only one set of each exercise. This will minimize muscular soreness, which is a common occurrence in the first week or two of training. After several weeks a decision can be made as to how rapidly you wish to gain strength and whether or not you are willing to spend extra time to perform three sets. One could perform three sets in the areas where strength is deficient, and in other movements one set could be performed. If you wish to maximize strength in certain movements, then performing six sets with heavy weights, which allows only four to eight repetitions per set, will result in a still greater strength stimulus. Such a program, however, should only be used by physically mature persons who have trained consistently over many months or years and who are willing to spend rather large amounts of time in strength building. Such a system is similar to the training programs used by competitive weight lifters in Olympic style and power lifting competition.

Repetitions and Load

The term "repetitions" refers to the number of movements made in one exercise in one set. Ten repetitions are completed when you have done ten push-ups, for example. The number of repetitions varies with the amount of resistance overcome. More repetitions can be done with light weights while the opposite is obviously true of heavier weights. Thus, weight and repetitions are inversely related.

Greater strength is developed as you progressively overload the neuromuscular system. For sheer strength, the best weight to select would theoretically be one that you can barely raise one time. This is not advocated because the safety hazard greatly increases. I prefer to use a range of repetitions when prescribing resistance training exercise rather than estimating a starting poundage for a given exercise. Quite honestly, the latter is just too difficult to do. Some books suggest use of a selected percentage of body weight but my experience suggests that body size is not a meaningful predictor of strength. A 120-pound cross-country runner may find that curls with a 75-pound barbell are heavy. He or she may struggle to do four or five repetitions, whereas a lineman on the football team may find 75 pounds light and may be able to do 15 to 20 repetitions with that load. Similarly, a 120-pound woman who emphasizes walking and aerobic dance in her exercise program may find that trying to perform the bench press with 60 pounds (half of her bodyweight) may be far too much, whereas a woman gymnast of the same weight but with a more compact body build and more muscle may find the same weight very appropriate or even too light.

To build strength rapidly and also safely, you should perform each exercise about 8 to 15 repetitions, and upon completing the last movement in each exercise, you should feel that an additional repetition would not have been possible. This range of repetitions provides an effective stimulus for strength as well as local muscle endurance development.

I do not feel there is one recommendation that can be made for all people as to how heavy the training load should be. For rapidly growing adolescents whose bone growth is incomplete, I wouldn't recommend lifting any load that can't be done for at least eight repetitions using strict technique. Many of the pulls, strains, and other injuries people experience while resistance training occur when the load becomes too heavy to move with good form. Consequently, in order to lift a load a bit heavier or to perform one more repetition with a heavy load, the body position tends to be altered. For example, the back is arched while doing a bench press, or the back is arched while trying to curl a barbell. The alteration in posture typically places undue strain on one or more joints, and injury results. Often the joint overload occurs to the lower back. Back problems are common enough without adding to them in a fitness program. They can also be debilitating, slow-healing injuries.

A second point to consider in selecting the load and repetitions is the relative importance of strength in your fitness program. While it may be highly important for a high school football player, it probably is of far less importance for the average adult. Since a good level of strength can be achieved with 8 to 15 repetitions, I don't feel the injury risk/strength benefit ratio using fewer repetitions and heavier loads is justified in nonathletes. Furthermore, maximizing strength is probably unwarranted in most sports. The sports requiring high strength levels are those involving contact and acceleration of a large mass such as a shot put or of the entire body (for example, sprinting and football). Most other sports probably don't depend largely on strength. For these latter activities, spending extra time lifting heavy weights not only may be dangerous but it may also be counterproductive. For example, additional body weight, even if it is largely muscle mass, may slow down a sprinter, fatigue an endurance athlete, and weigh down a gymnast. Note that even the participants in most Olympic events, basketball and volleyball included, do not possess the bulky musculature of the superenthused weight trainer or body builder. It seems that in most sporting events, a little bit of muscle goes a long way. I do feel, however, that all athletes should develop and then maintain a reasonable level of strength to reduce injury potential and to remove any weak links that may otherwise limit their performance. This principle is just as applicable to females as it is to males.

Specificity of Strength

Strength is developed primarily in those movements or lifts specifically practiced. This training principle is known as specificity of strength. The best way to increase your strength in an exercise is to train with that particular exercise. Although such a statement seems obvious and common sense, it is worth emphasizing. It is too easy to generalize about strength. You could observe someone performing a 300- or 400-pound bench press and believe that person would be stronger than others in other exercises as well. People often develop a particular liking for one or two exercises and consequently do many sets of these exercises while neglecting others. They develop a high level of strength in these specific exercises but their overall general strength will not be similarly developed. To optimize the development of muscular fitness in general, one will do best to utilize a wide variety of general weight training exercises and develop strength in many movements and muscles. Athletes, in addition to performing general exercises, should also perform some exercises that mimic the actual movements inherent in the sport. For example, pole vaulters often do pull-ups in the inverted position because this is the position in which they must pull while actually pole vaulting. Similarly, basketball and volleyball players typically do jumping exercises with light weights to enhance their jumping power.

Do Not Hold the Breath While Lifting

If you lift weights while holding your breath, considerable pressure is developed within the chest cavity. The pressure can be strong enough to clamp shut large veins in the chest, which reduces the return of blood to the heart. In addition, arteries taking blood from the heart to the tissues are squeezed and narrowed. These changes result in a reduction of blood flow from the heart. Symptoms such as light-headedness, dizziness, and seeing bright lights or even blacking out may occur. To minimize the development of pressure in the chest while lifting, you should keep the airways open by vigorously forcing air out of the lungs as you perform each repetition. This can be done by making a grunting noise while you expire. The harder you work or contract your muscles, the harder you should expire. Normally, people inspire while lifting a weight and expire while lowering it. So, as long as air is continually passing out of the airways, high pressure buildup in the chest can be avoided. The other factor that increases the likelihood of being affected by this condition is the length of time the airway is closed. If you strained to lift a heavy weight for 5 to 10 seconds as a competitive weight lifter might during a maximal lift, then the reduction of blood flow is prolonged, increasing the likelihood of the symptoms appearing.

Contraindications for Weight Training

If you have high blood pressure or any form of heart disease, check with your physician prior to doing any resistance training. Blood pressure is elevated significantly even at relatively modest levels of tension development. As skeletal muscles contract, they squeeze blood vessels running through them. At about 60% of one's peak strength, arteries in the upper extremity are almost totally squeezed shut. In the lower extremities this occurs at about 75% of the maximum strength. As the heart beats and forces blood into temporarily blocked vessels, the pressure inside the vessels rises dramatically.

Typically, heart patients are advised not to perform isometric (muscle contractions that produce no movement) or vigorous sustained contractions because the elevated pressure within the arteries may be dangerously high, and because the workload on the heart is greatly increased due to the building pressure against which the heart has to work. The increased effort required by a diseased heart muscle or limited coronary circulation to the heart may be expressed by a symptom such as chest pain and/or pressure (angina pectoris). Blood pressure in competitive weight lifters while they are actually lifting has been measured at over 400 mm Hg systolic and 300 mm Hg diastolic (while at rest the normal range of blood pressure is 100 to 140 for systolic pressure and 60 to 90 for diastolic pressure). This represents an extreme pressure overload on the heart as well as the vessels and at this time, it is unknown if there are ill effects that may occur over years of such activity. For those with elevated blood pressure or a heart condition, however, resistance training should most likely be limited. If such a person is permitted to do strength work, it should be of moderate or even low intensity and consist of rhythmic effort rather than sustained or isometric contractions.

Periodic Change

When progress in muscular fitness has stopped, alter the training program. Strength and local muscle endurance are components of fitness that can be easily and readily improved.

Most people who have never trained with weights or resistance-type exercise are able to demonstrate excellent progress in the first month or two of training. If performing only selected exercises, which develop many muscle groups simultaneously, as suggested here, the cost in terms of time and energy are quite small. However, at some point, everyone reaches a plateau of performance, and further progress can be made only by working harder. The whole idea of building strength is dependent on the progressive nature of the overload or stimulus. As long as one presents a stronger training stimulus to the neuromuscular and skeletal systems, and if adequate recovery is allowed between training sessions so that the tissues can supercompensate physiologically, then strength and local endurance will continually increase, at least in theory.

What every weight trainer eventually learns is that slight alteration of the training stimulus allows you to train with greater intensity for several weeks, which signals further nerve, muscle, tendon and bone development. Let's assume you are a woman who weighs 140 pounds and your goal is to bench press 70 pounds 10 times but you seem unable to progress past 60 pounds with nine repetitions. Training could be modified to consist of 40 or 50 pounds with 3 sets of as many repetitions as possible. Using a bit heavier weight than my target weight on one training session followed by the use of a lighter weight on the next session has worked nicely for me over the years. By the third scheduled session with the target weight of 60 pounds, quite likely you will make the 10 repetitions of 60 pounds or even more and be ready to progress to 65 or 70 pounds.

Most people who have trained with weights over a period of years modify their training regimen quite frequently, suggesting that variation in training may be fundamental to adhering to training. You could lift relatively heavier weights 1 day each week while using light and moderate loads the other 2 days, or you could use an entirely different series of exercises once each week.

Kids and Weight Training

At what age should adolescents begin resistance or weight training? This is a question I am often asked by parents and youngsters of youth sport teams I coach. The pat answer given by medical and physical education authorities has been that overstrenuous strength training in children and adolescents may damage the growth centers of the long bones in the extremities. I think authorities making such advice have had to be conservative to discourage overzealous parents, coaches and adolescents from doing excessive training that could lead to early closure of the growth center, thereby stopping growth of the long bones. However, it is difficult if not impossible to define "excessive" training as it would undoubtedly vary among youngsters. Variation in body weight and maturation make it ridiculous to identify a specific weight that is possibly damaging. Common sense must predominate if a sound decision is to be made.

I don't mean to suggest from these comments that children should never vigorously exercise; far from it! Fitness levels of many American children are too low today. Fitness and medical authorities urge that all children should engage in vigorous activity for 1 hour daily. Many children do not meet this recommendation. Healthy children naturally seem to want to play vigorous games, but few have the desire to do so in a structured type of exercise such as weight training. What's more, children active in a wide variety of games and sport are able to develop all components of fitness simultaneously, but in addition they are developing skills in a multitude of body movements. Also, they have a great time doing it. Contrast such diverse training to the drudgery to which we adults often subject ourselves. The notion of counting laps while running or swimming or counting the number of calisthenics one does probably never occurs to children. They move vigorously and continuously except for frequent pauses to recover and rebuild their energy supply. Some of my most enjoyable, yet vigorous, workouts have been playing with my own children and their friends.

Researchers have only recently begun to investigate the extent to which children are trainable. While active children will possess greater fitness including better muscular strength and endurance than less-active children, it appears that the magnitude of change resulting from training is less in children. Several studies have shown that children or adolescents become more trainable about one year after they have passed their phase of greatest growth in height and weight. The age at which peak height gain occurs varies widely in children, but studies indicate that at age 12 to 13, adolescents are able to significantly gain strength with training. However, I still think it is best to delay formal resistance training for a while. I would rather see youngsters building strength and endurance as a result of participation in a wide variety of vigorous activities such as climbing, sprinting, bicycling, soccer, swimming, basketball, baseball, gymnastics, and skiing. Children who have a rich background in many activities usually wind up more skilled in selected sports once they are in junior and senior high school. Possession of numerous skills should increase the likelihood of being active and fit as an adult. Perhaps all youth activities should be examined in light of the effect they may have later in life. Even if one was attempting to produce champion athletes, I believe the emphasis on diversity of activity, and total physical fitness and skill, would be a better means of training than having children and young adolescents overemphasize strength development. I also know quite a few dads who have bought their sons barbells and accessory equipment at young ages only to find that the equipment is not used much after several sessions. As stated previously, strength can be developed quickly. I don't think potential athletes will fall behind others because of not training with weights. Because of the reasons discussed here I favor holding off on the formal strength training until about age 14 or 15.

Basic Strength Exercises

One means of making sure that most of the large muscles receive a training effect is to select exercises that activate many of the major muscles simultaneously. Many books recommend doing a large number of exercises each training session. However, it has been my experience that most people don't have the time to do 15, 20, or 25 separate exercises. Also, for most people, I believe it is more important for health to spend enough time exercising to develop aerobic fitness. I recommend to most people that it is better to exercise 30 minutes 3 times weekly to gain the benefits associated with aerobic activities than it is to reduce this time in order to spend much of their exercise time on muscular fitness. If you have the time and motivation to spend several hours each week weight training, that's fine, but beyond a point the extra time taken will likely not result in better health. Consequently, a system I have found effective is to group exercises according to the major muscles they develop. This results in four groups of exercises I refer to as the Big Four, which are summarized in Table 7.

This classification of exercises allows you to train most of the large muscles by performing one exercise from each group. In terms of time, this is an efficient way to develop and maintain muscular fitness. Furthermore, if these exercises are done following an aerobic training session, then the time needed for warm-up is reduced. I use this sequence and find that when I reach the weight room after a run, I only need some light calisthenics such as a set of push-ups and sit-ups before proceeding directly into my first set of each weight exercise. My first set of each exercise, however, is still a light one. I do a second set of exercises that relate to my fitness goals at that time. For example, in the winter when I play basketball several days each week, I do a second set of quadriceps (muscles in the front of the thigh) exercises, which helps my jumping and rebounding. This limited but efficient approach to muscular fitness keeps a person in a continual state of read-

Table 7 Classification of Exercises for Muscular Fitness (The Big Four)

Category	Exercises	Major muscles developed
Push	Bench press	Pectoralis major & minor Triceps Deltoids
	Sitting press	Triceps Deltoids Trapezius
	Push-ups	Same as bench press
Pull	Rowing motion	Latissimus dorsi Triceps Biceps Teres major & minor Subscupularis Supra- and infraspinatus Rhomboids
	Lat pull	Same as rowing motion
	Pull-ups	Same as rowing motion
Abdominals	Pelvic tilt	Rectus abdominus Internal & external oblique
	Trunk curl	Same as pelvic tilt
	Trunk rotation	Same as pelvic tilt
Hip and thigh	Half-squat	Quadriceps Glutei Hamstrings
	Knee extension	Quadriceps
	Bench or stair stepping	Same as half-squat

iness for sports, work around the house, and provides one with a feeling of pep, power and limb lightness when walking up stairs, playing with the kids and in general, living an active life.

There is a specific reason for the inclusion of the abdominal exercise group in the Big Four. Possession of good abdominal strength and endurance provides protection to the lower back. If the abdominal muscles are relatively weak in comparison to the lower back muscles and hip flexor muscles (the latter are located in the front of the hip and thigh), the pelvis is tilted forward. This increases the curvature in the lower back, which increases the pressure on spinal nerves adjacent to the spinal column. The discs of cartilage between each segment of the spinal column are filled with thick, syrupy fluid. When the lower back curve is increased, the spine squeezes the discs backward and laterally. As the discs bulge outward and sideward they exert pressure on the spinal nerves, causing pain. The pain produces contraction or spasm of surrounding muscles, which makes the back stiff as well as painful. Consequently, the abdominal muscles should be strengthened to withstand the tendency of the back muscles to tilt the pelvis forward. Furthermore, because even the normal spine has a curve in the lower back, there is a tendency for gravity to tilt the pelvis and exert greater compression of the lower back. This is why prolonged standing and sitting can elicit lower back discomfort. In addition to strengthening the abdominal muscles, good care of the lower back requires maintenance of flexibility in the muscles that tilt the pelvis forward. These muscles include the hip flexors, hamstrings, and lower back muscles. Exercises to stretch these muscle groups are discussed in the next chapter.

The following figures illustrate the exercises listed in Table 7. A description of each exercise is provided here.

Pushing Exercises

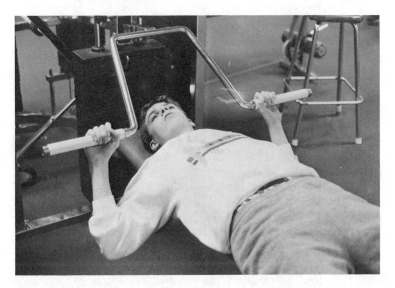

Bench press. Lying on the back, tighten the abdominal muscles and push the lower back into the bench. Keep the lower back in this position throughout the exercise to prevent it from being arched. Push the bar directly overhead; lower until the bar touches the chest and repeat. Most people use a grip with the hands placed about shoulder-width apart. However, one can alter the hand spacing and modify the extent to which various muscles are stimulated. A narrower grip places more emphasis on the triceps muscles of the back and side of the arms and a lesser emphasis is placed on the chest muscles (pectoralis major and minor). A wider grip has the opposite effect.

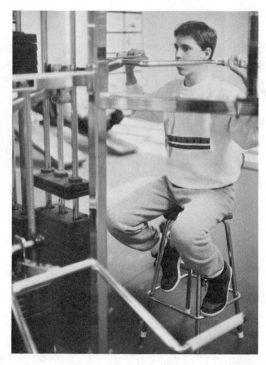

Sitting press. It is recommended that exercises that involve pushing weights overhead should not be done while standing because the lower back usually becomes arched while pushing a weight overhead. Consequently, it tends to produce back discomfort and tightness. If performed while sitting, the arching of the lower back is minimized. However, to prevent any arching of the back the abdominal muscles should be tensed isometrically throughout the upward portion of the lift. This may divert part of your attention while learning to tense two muscle groups simultaneously, but once learned, it will offer considerable protection to the back.

An additional factor that helps to minimize arching of the back when sitting or standing is to look directly ahead while raising the bar rather than watching the bar. When you look at the bar, the back of the neck as well as the lower back become arched. A shoulder-width grip is generally recommended but the hand spacing will vary the training effect. A wider grip works the shoulders to a greater extent and the triceps to a lesser extent. A narrower spacing has the opposite effect.

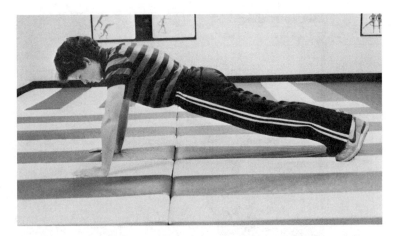

Figure 1 Push-up

Push-ups.   The standard push-up is a simple yet excellent developmental exercise for a large number of muscles. A strict push-up (Figure 1) begins with touching the chest to the floor and pushing until the elbows are fully straight. The back should be keep straight, which requires tensing the abdominal muscles and muscles of the buttocks. Have someone watch you do the exercise so that you can correctly maintain the desired position. To avoid tightening the back of the neck, tuck the chin towards the chest throughout the exercise. If unable to perform the push-up as described above, bend your knees and let them remain on the floor. This alteration reduces the total weight you must lift and therefore makes it possible for people with an initially lower level of arm-shoulder muscular fitness to use this exercise. Another means of making the exercise easier is to perform the movement against a wall (Figure 2). The exercise becomes more difficult as the feet are placed progressively further from the wall. To make push-ups more advanced or difficult one may elevate the feet as seen in Figure 3. Further progression can be achieved by moving the feet to a greater height.

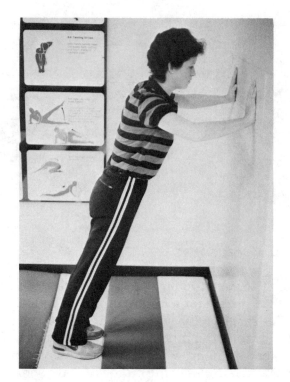

Figure 2 Wall push-up

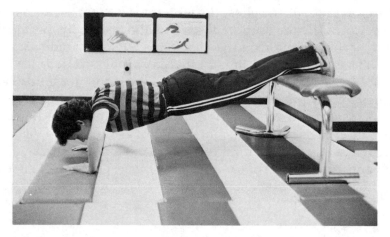

Figure 3 Advanced push-up

Pulling Exercises

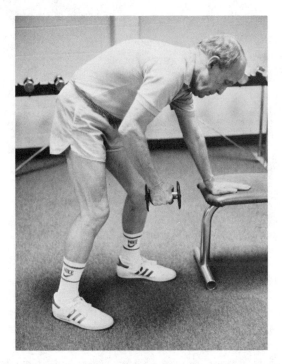

Rowing motion. I recommend doing this exercise with a dumbbell rather than a barbell, because it reduces the strain on the lower back. By placing one hand on a bench or chair, even less strain is placed on the spine. Raise the dumbbell until it is as high as the chest or until it touches the shoulder. Lower the weight and lightly touch the floor before raising it again.

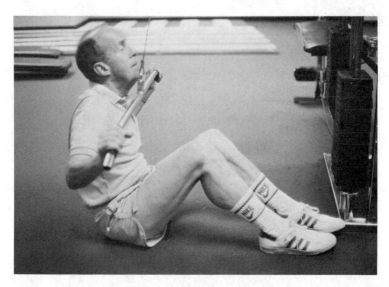

Lat pull.   This exercise is shown performed on a Universal Gym. The bar is pulled down to the chest or behind the head to the shoulders, or these movements may be alternated. The former movement emphasizes development of the latissimus dorsi, the large muscle beneath the armpit, while the latter movement emphasizes development of the upper back musculature, such as the trapezius, rhomboids and posterior deltoids.

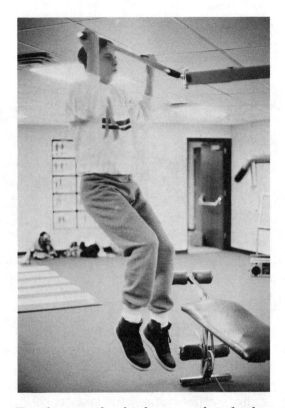

Pull-ups. For those with a high strength to body weight ratio this exercise is nearly identical to the lat pull exercise except the body is pulled up to the bar instead of the bar being pulled down to the body. The exercise can be made a bit easier by gripping the bar with the palms facing you. This hand position also favors a better development of the biceps. For advanced trainers, a weight can be attached to a belt or pinched between the legs.

Abdominal Exercises

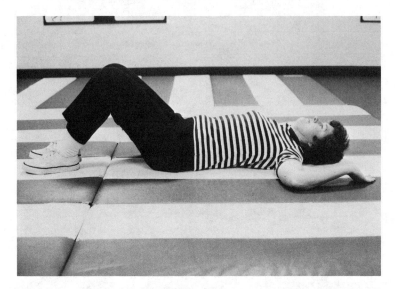

Pelvic tilt.   Lie on the floor with the knees bent. Tighten the abdominal wall and push the lower back firmly against the floor; hold several seconds and relax. Progress in this exercise by sustaining each isometric contraction for a longer time and/or doing more repetitions. This is a good beginning abdominal exercise.

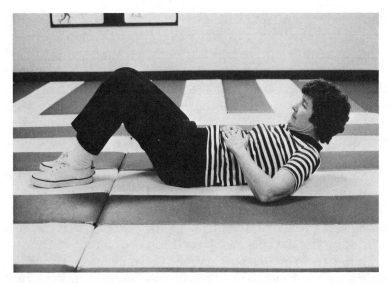

Trunk curl. This exercise has become the classic one to develop the abdominal musculature without placing strain on the lower back. The movement is to be done slowly in two separate movements. The chin is first tucked to the chest while the shoulders are barely raised off the floor. Then the spinal column is slowly flexed so that each vertebra is raised in sequence. The upward movement is stopped at about 30°; any further elevation is accomplished largely by the frontal hip muscles which, because of their attachment to the lumbar vertebrae, tend to cause lower back discomfort. The downward movement should be equally slow and should also proceed vertebra by vertebra. This is radically different from the arm-flapping, straight-leg sit-ups people used to do. Note that the feet are not anchored under anything such as a barbell or sofa. Anchoring the feet allows the hip flexors to do much of the work, which reduces the relative contribution and the training effect of the abdominals. For this reason, trunk curls performed with the feet anchored, including sit-ups on a slant board, are not recommended.

An additional difference in this trunk curl exercise as compared to most of the older abdominal exercises is that the hips and knees are bent throughout the movement. The bent joint positions shorten the muscles that cross them. When muscles are shortened, their capacity to produce tension decreases. In this case it is the frontal hip muscles that are purposely shortened, which then places more of the load on the abdominals. The second reason for assuming this position is that it reduces the ballast effect of the legs and pelvis. That is, when the legs are left straight out to the front, the long lever exerts more of an anchoring effect on the feet. When the abdominals contract to raise the trunk, the greater the ballast or inertia of the lower extremity, and the less the tension required by the abdominals to raise the upper extremity. Thus, the degree of difficulty in performing the trunk curl will depend largely on the degree to which the hips and knees are bent. If you have never done the exercise as described, you may find that you are unable to do even a single repetition correctly. A good way to start the exercise is to perform just the first phase or just raise the head and shoulders, and hold the position for 2 seconds. You can progress by doing more repetitions of this first phase. Realize that the abdominals are being strengthened, although the end position of 30° is not achieved. After several weeks most people are able to perform the 30° movement with the knees partially bent. As the abdominals become further strengthened, the exercise can be done with the knees more fully bent.

Another means of making the trunk curl progressive is to vary the position of the arms. The exercise is easiest to do when the hands are placed on the abdominal wall or beside the hips on the floor. To make the movement more difficult, cross the arms on the chest. The next progression is to clasp the hands behind the head. Once able to perform the exercise strictly and slowly about 10 times with the hands behind the head, you have achieved a high level of abdominal strength and muscle endurance, and so have provided considerable protection to the lower back.

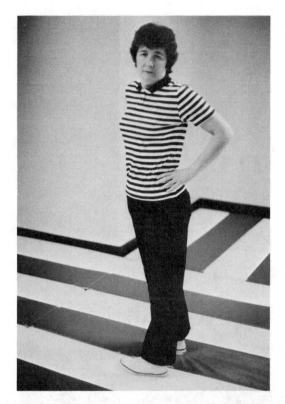

Trunk rotation. While sucking in the abdominal wall and keeping the pelvis up, slowly rotate the trunk as far as possible to the right. Return to the front and while sustaining the tension in the abdominal wall, rotate slowly to the left. Do not hold the breath but breathe continuously. Progress by doing more repetitions, sucking in harder, and twisting farther.

Hip and Thigh Exercises

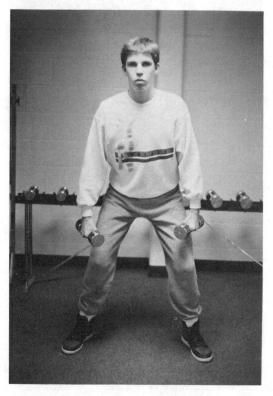

Half-squat.   This is the classic exercise for the quadriceps. The feet should be placed about shoulder-width apart. A barbell is typically placed behind the head resting on the shoulders but I feel this jeopardizes the lower back. I recommend holding a weight in each hand because with a barbell on the shoulders, balance is precarious and far more strain is placed on the lower back. Lower yourself, under control, until the knees are at about a 100° position or until the thighs begin to approach a position parallel to the ground. Any further lowering tends to stretch the knee ligaments, reducing the stability of the knee. Also, the more the knees are bent the more the pressure placed on the kneecap. If you have knee problems be extremely cautious with this or any other knee bending exercise. I usually only lower my body to a comfortable semi-crouch position. Few of us need strength in a deeper position.

The entire upward and downward portions of the lift should be performed with the back as erect as possible. Competitive weight lifters often focus on an object directly in front of them that they contend assists in keeping the back straight. It is important to keep the spine straight to reduce pressure on the spinal discs and nerves. Throughout the exercise, keep the pelvis in a tucked-in position to protect the lower back.

It is interesting to note that the results of a recent photographic analysis of elite power lifters indicated that the best lifters in the squat maintained a more erect posture than the lesser lifters while performing the lift. It may be that the more erect position allows more effective use of the quadricep muscles of the frontal thigh as well as the posterior muscles of the thigh and hip (that is, the hamstrings and gluteus maximus). It certainly is a safer way to lift, which may reduce injuries in weight trainers and lifters. It may be that the better athletes lift this way to avoid injury, which in turn makes them better lifters.

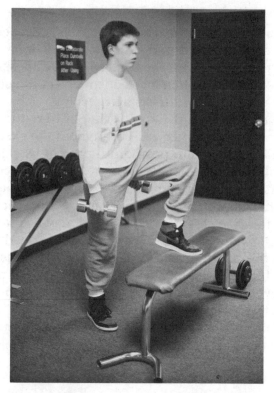

Bench or stair stepping.   A sturdy bench or chair is needed
for this exercise. The movement consists simply of stepping
up and down. The knee of the stepping leg should be fully
straightened once atop the bench to ensure development of
the inner portion of the quadriceps muscle, the vastus medialis. Once you progress beyond lifting just your body weight,
additional weight used in this exercise should be held at hip
height, for example, by holding two dumbbells or a barbell.
The rationale for this is to reduce the strain on the lower back.
Anytime a load is carried above the waist, such as when
placing a barbell across the back of the shoulders, there is an
increased tendency to arch the lower back and to later suffer
tightness, spasm, and aching. The exercise is done with one
leg a given number of repetitions and then repeated with the
opposite leg.

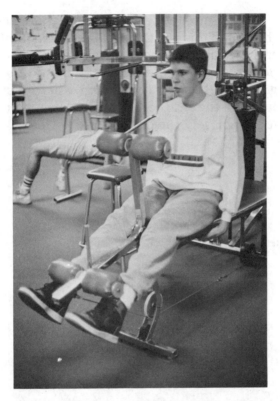

Knee extension.   From a starting position with the knees bent, the legs are raised until the knees are fully straightened. Failure to completely straighten the joints results in a lesser development of the inner portion of the quadriceps called the vastus medialis. To maximize development of the vastus medialis, hold the knee straight for each repetition for one or two counts. Whereas most people completely lower the foot to begin each repetition, I recommend lowering the foot only about one third of the way down. This will reduce knee strain. When the knee is more fully bent the kneecap is compressed into the joint tissues with considerable force. Consequently, many people experience pain and inflammation after doing this exercise. To reduce this tendency, one should avoid lifting in the first portion of the lift except, of course, for the first repetition. Because most activities do not require bending the knees much beyond this position, the somewhat limited range of movement still builds strength and endurance in the normal range of motion. While this exercise is an excellent one for developing the quadriceps, it works no other muscle group. It should be noted that the half-squat and bench or stair step exercise works not only the quadriceps but also the gluteals and hamstrings.

chapter 8

Flexibility

Flexibility is an important aspect of fitness for a number of reasons. Inadequate flexibility may lead to muscle pulls. These injuries occur not only to young athletes but to the middle-aged and elderly as well. Most of us have probably experienced muscle pulls and the associated discomfort. Many pulls occur during relatively light exercise or work, which indicates that inflexible joints pose a hazard during many daily activities. Therefore, even if you do not plan on participating in strenuous sports, a stretching program is beneficial.

Flexibility typically is reduced with aging particularly in those who are sedentary. The reasons are twofold. One is that the connective tissues such as bone, cartilage, tendon, and ligament lose some of the protein that provides elasticity to these tissues. Secondly, connective tissues become tighter with prolonged inactivity. For example, even a child loses considerable flexibility if a limb is injured, placed in a sling, and kept immobile. Many middle-aged and elderly people are affected by both factors. The exact stimulus to maintain optimal flexibility is unknown but it is well understood that movements that allow the joint to be moved comfortably through the entire range of motion are effective in improving flexibility.

Normal flexibility enhances effective movement in daily tasks as well as in sports. A muscle-bound weight lifter is a good example. If he or she trained with weights or other muscle building devices and did not move the limbs through a wide range of motion while lifting, and also did no stretching, it is possible that he or she would lose flexibility. Many coaches and athletes have seen some individuals become overzealous about strength work and if they didn't stretch, they became less effective players although possessing greater size and strength. The importance of good flexibility in athletes is obvious in a principle of physics known as impulse. Impulse is the time over which a force acts, and the greater the time the greater the impulse that results in the production of greater speed. For example, compare two baseball pitchers: one with tight, inflexible shoulders and the other with normally flexible shoulders. If they produce the same muscle force, the flexible pitcher would release the ball with greater velocity simply because of having more time to accelerate the pitching arm. Athletes throw farther, kick farther and run faster largely because of good flexibility in the related joints. If such an athlete correctly improves his or her strength, then an outstanding performer may be produced.

Good athletes are often good models of effective, efficient human movement. Their grace, smoothness, and rhythm are in part attributed to their excellent flexibility. Lack of flexibility, on the other hand, makes us appear older than we really are as well as less efficient. I've often wondered how many traffic accidents are caused by people with inflexible spinal columns who are unable to rotate the spine to allow them to quickly and easily look behind them prior to changing lanes while driving. Even the energy cost of moving our joints is reduced by maintaining good flexibility. You don't see many tight, stiff-moving athletes. These characteristics are incongruous with efficient movement.

A major cause of aches and pains in people is tightened muscles. Shortened, overly tense muscles can alter the position of bones meeting at a joint, thus altering posture. Lower backache is one of the most common complaints and also is a leading cause of job absenteeism, reduced productivity, and increased medical costs. The most common cause of the problem is strength and flexibility imbalance. The abdominal muscles tend to be weak while the lower back muscles and those of the frontal hip region and hamstrings are tightened. Appropriate stretching can often correct this problem. No one moves efficiently if their muscles or joints are tight and painful. If these conditions exist for long, they can alter posture and limit the ease, efficiency, and comfort of movement.

Unfortunately, many people do not realize how effective exercise can be in reducing the problem. Consequently, they endure the discomfort and reduced efficiency for many years.

Testing and Developing Your Flexibility

Because flexibility is not a general trait, assessment of it should include measures at several of the large joints where tightness is common. A number of tests are described and illustrated here so that you can assess the extent of your flexibility. Each test is also an effective stretching exercise for the given region. Before stretching be sure to thoroughly warm up with at least 5 minutes of light aerobic exercise.

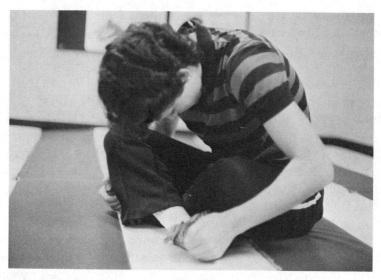

Lower Back

Sit cross-legged and slowly bend forward as low as comfortably possible. Acceptable flexibility should allow your nose to come within 8 inches of the floor.

Tight lower back muscles frequently cause an increase in the curvature of the lower back, which increases pressure on the vertebral discs. These discs act as shock absorbers for the spinal column but when excess pressure is placed on them, they are partly squeezed out of place and can irritate adjacent spinal nerves. Therefore, a key component in care of the lower back includes stretching of the back muscles to prevent or reduce this excess curvature.

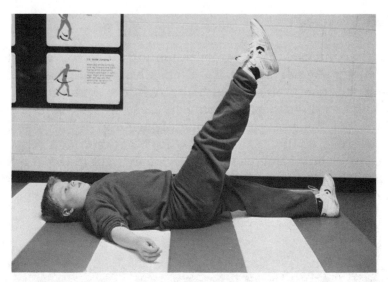

Hamstrings (Muscles Running the Length of the Back of the Thigh)

Lie with legs straight and keep the lower back flat on the floor. Raise one leg slowly as far as comfortably possible with the knee held straight. A decent score is reaching a position where the thigh and leg are nearly vertical; reaching vertical is a good score while movement beyond vertical (beyond 90°) is a superior score.

Adequate hamstring flexibility is important in preventing lower back pain. Like the lower back muscles, tightened hamstrings exert a forward and downward pull on the pelvis, which increases the lumbar or lower back curvature. For athletes, good flexibility in these muscles is critical in terms of preventing hamstring pulls while sprinting. A number of studies have found that the limb in which hamstring pulls occur tends to be tighter than its counterpart.

Calf Muscles

Two muscles, the gastrocnemius and the soleus, comprise the major mass of the calf. If it is inflexible, you are more likely to experience problems with the Achilles tendon (such as Achilles tendinitis), which connects these muscles to the back of the foot. Such problems frequently occur in people past age 30 who overdo their exercise or who do not thoroughly warm up. For example, joggers are notoriously tight in this tendon unless they regularly stretch. However, even hikers, dancers, and rope jumpers use these muscles extensively and are prone to tightness here.

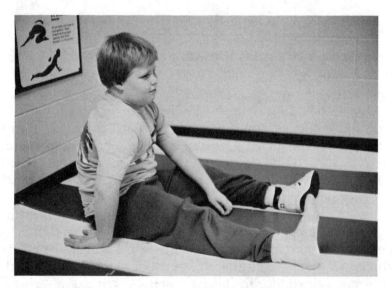

Gastrocnemius. Sit with one knee straight and using the muscles in the front of the leg, bend the foot toward the knee. The normal range of motion is about 15° to 20° past vertical.

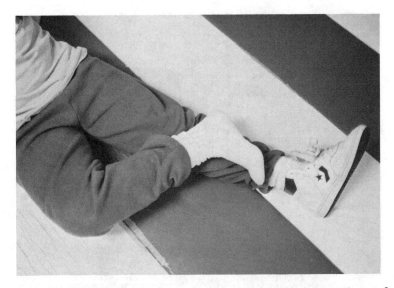

Soleus. This flexibility test is identical to the one above for the gastrocnemius except the knee is bent. You should strive to eventually bend the foot toward the knee about 15° to 20° past the neutral position (position of the foot while standing on a flat surface).

While both of the above tests are effective to evaluate flexibility of the calf, they are not particularly effective as stretching exercises because they don't allow an adequate stretching force to be exerted. The following two exercises are commonly used by joggers, walkers, dancers and other athletes to stretch these two muscles.

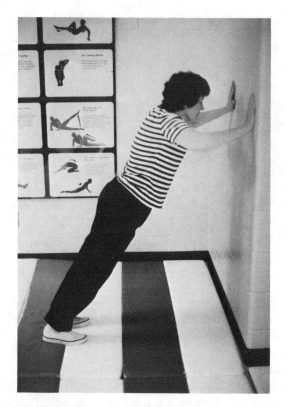

Gastrocnemius. Walk up to a wall or fence and place the feet straight ahead and about 18 inches from the wall. Place the hands on the wall, and with the entire body held straight, bend forward as far as comfortably possible. Throughout the movement the heels must maintain firm contact with the ground; if they are raised, the stretch on these muscles and their common tendon is reduced. If no real stretch is felt with the feet at the starting position, move the feet back several inches. As your flexibility improves the feet are moved progressively farther from the wall.

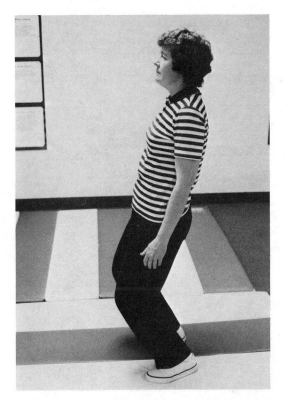

Soleus.   Hold a chair or some object close by and bend both knees while keeping the heels on the ground. Slowly bend down until a comfortable stretch is felt in the Achilles tendon and hold this position. Maintaining this semi-squat position will tax the frontal thigh muscles (quadriceps). If they tire easily, do a series of stretches each held for several seconds.

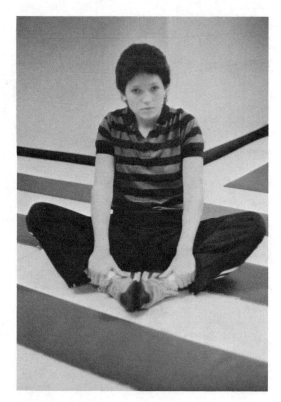

Groin or Inner Thigh

Sit on the floor with the soles of the feet touching. Lower the outside of each knee as far as you can comfortably go. A good range of motion in these muscles will allow the outer knee to come within about 6 inches from the floor when the feet are placed about 1 foot from the buttocks.

Groin tightness can pose a problem in athletes who sprint, dance, and jump. Muscle pulls are all too common here and can remove an athlete from practice or competition. So, particularly for athletes, good flexibility of the groin muscles is important in injury prevention.

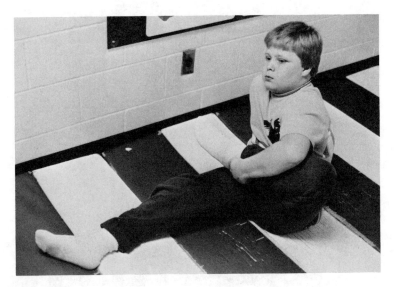

Outer Hip

While sitting, grasp the outer foot and outer calf. Gently bring the thigh toward your chest. A good score in this test is bringing the calf within 6 inches from the chest while you are sitting upright.

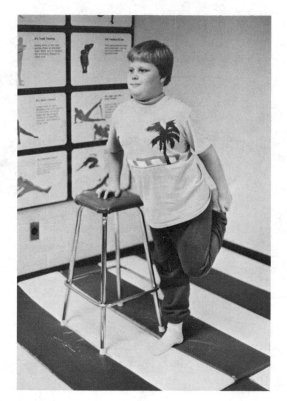

Frontal Hip

Stand and hold a chair or table for balance. Bend one foot backwards and grasp it with the hand on the same side. Point the knee directly at the ground and keep it in this position throughout the stretch. While standing erect, gently and slowly lift the foot with your hand until the foot touches your derriere or as high as can comfortably be done. Good flexibility here should allow you to bring the foot within several inches from the buttocks.

Tightness in this area promotes lower back problems because these muscles attach to the lumbar vertebrae. Consequently, they exert a forward pull on the lower back, which increases the curve in the lumbar spine. This in turn increases pressure on the vertebral discs and adjacent spinal nerves.

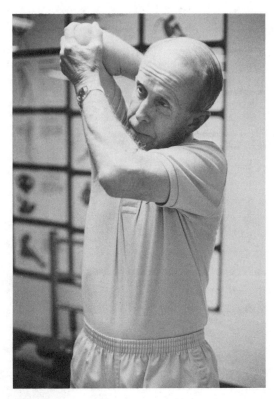

Shoulder Extensors

Raise one elbow as high as possible while touching the shoulder on the same side. Gently push the elbow up with the other hand attempting to raise the elbow as high as comfortably possible. Adequate flexibility will let you raise the arm until the elbow is pointed directly overhead.

Adequate flexibility in these muscles allows for a normal positioning of the shoulders, which enhances posture. Tightness here affects sport performance by limiting the extent and ease with which the arms can be moved overhead and backward. For example, the backswing in the tennis serve or forehand would be reduced by inflexibility, as would a windup before throwing.

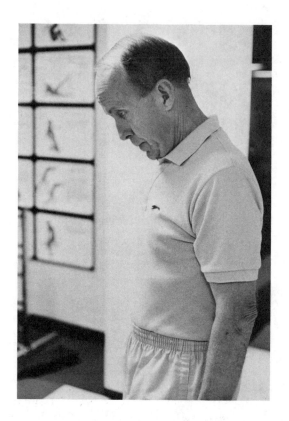

Neck

Slowly lower the chin until it touches the upper chest. Slowly drag the chin across the upper right chest progressing as far as you can comfortably go. Repeat to the left. Good flexibility will allow you to look directly to the side when at the end position.

Another effective stretching exercise for the neck is a slow rotation of the neck in each direction. Begin with the chin on the chest and take a full 10 seconds to complete one revolution. Do not move the head backwards while circling as it tends to compress cervical nerves and create tightness and soreness in the back of the neck. Repeat in the other direction. This really feels good when you have been sitting for prolonged periods and your neck muscles get stiff and tense.

By assessing your flexibility at each major joint you can determine what areas need most attention. As previously mentioned, you may find that your backache, sore shoulder, or stiff neck becomes less bothersome. I would recommend performing one exercise for each muscle group listed at least three times each week and 5 or more days a week for areas where you are tight.

How to Stretch

Until the 1960s nearly everyone stretched by repetitive bouncing. Researchers, however, observed that every time a muscle is stretched quickly, it stimulates nerve endings in the muscle, which are sensitive to stretch. They cause the muscle to contract reflexively, which means that while one stretches, the tension in the muscle increases, resisting the stretching motion. Consequently, such jerky-type bouncing may cause small tears in the connective tissue. Current stretching techniques used by physical educators and physical therapists employ a slow and gradual lengthening followed by holding the end point for a period of 10 to 60 seconds. The muscles stretched in this manner are more relaxed, which should allow a better and safer lengthening of the connective tissues.

Another stretching technique that is becoming popular involves an alternation of stretching and contracting of a muscle or muscle group. It is called proprioceptive neuromuscular facilitation or PNF. Figure 8 demonstrates how the limb is first moved to a point of mild resistance or where slight discomfort occurs. The limb is held in the position while the stretched muscle is isometrically contracted. An isometric contraction is one in which the muscle(s) is tensed but the limb is not moved. The contraction is followed by a second slow stretch to a new point of mild tightness or resistance and here again the muscle(s) is isometrically contracted. This procedure continues until the limb or joint cannot be further moved

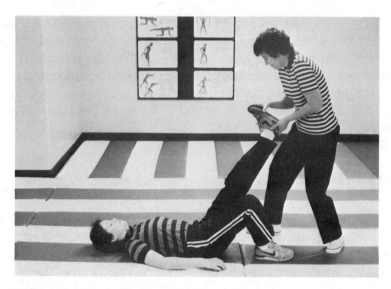

Figure 8   PNF stretching

comfortably. Both of these techniques rely on the pain threshold of the individual and it is emphasized that stretching should not be painful. Pain generally is the manner the nervous system uses to communicate overload; ignoring such a warning does not seem wise. Several studies have compared the slow stretch technique with the PNF stretch and found the latter to be more effective.

A new concept in stretching concerns when it should be performed. Traditionally, stretching is done at the very onset of exercise. Recent evidence, however, suggests that the most effective time to enhance the lengthening of connective tissue is when it is heated. The major protein in connective tissue, collagen, becomes softer and more pliable when heated; this is why a long period of cooking will soften even the toughest of meats. So, if you are stretching to improve flexibility, the main reason for stretching, it is probably most efficient to do so after some period of exercise. Many athletes today warm up by tossing a ball, slowly jogging, or doing some similar activity for a period and then doing their stretching. I stretch very briefly before a workout but afterward I devote 5 to 10 minutes to a thorough and longer stretch for the major muscle groups. My warm-up is in part governed by the nature of the activity. If my warm-up is running, then I run slowly until I perceive a smoothness and efficiency in my muscles, joints and breathing, then I gradually pick up the pace. Even prior to competitive running I use this procedure. By gradually building up to the speed and intensity at which I anticipate working, I feel my body and mind are fully prepared for the work ahead. My serious stretching is done at the end of the vigorous activity when the temperature of the connective tissues is probably at maximum; it makes sense to me, feels right and has pretty much allowed me to exercise injury-free for many years.

chapter 9

Weight Control

The millions of dollars and millions of frustrating moments people spend in the Western World on the problem of obesity is incredible. Approximately one third of the American population is considered overweight with about half of these classified as obese, meaning they weigh 20% or more than the norm for their age, sex, and height. In our laboratory, we have found that about 10% to 12% of elementary school boys and girls are overweight. Yet, I watch the TV news showing the Afghanistan rebels hike through the foothills of the Himalayas continuing their struggle against the Russian invaders. The Afghans are lean; many Westerners would even call them skinny. We have a number of Afghan students at our university and they are also lean. The dean of our foreign studies department lived in Afghanistan for several years and informs me that they are an active people. They walk and bicycle in amounts we think only done by athletes. They eat a diet high in carbohydrates such as bread and rice and relatively low in protein and fat. This type of diet and expenditure of energy in physical activity is not unique, however, to the people of Afghanistan; nor is their leanness. The great majority of the world's population living outside the West, that is, the Third World nations, are lean people. Examine pictures taken during the Civil War and the early part of the 20th century. We used to be a population of lean people, yet people actually consumed more calories in those days.

Obesity seems to be increasing in the United States. Adults today average about 4 pounds heavier than people in 1960. What will happen in the next 25 years? In nonobese children the number of fat cells increases in the first 2 years of life and is stable until puberty when the number increases again. If excessive fat is deposited during these times that fat cells increase in number, additional fat cells are produced. The number of fat cells seems to explain why obese children find it difficult to lose weight when they become adults. After the age of 25, men and women gain about 1 pound each year while they lose about one fourth of a pound of lean tissue, mostly muscle and bone. The net gain then is 1.25 pounds of fat per year. It's no wonder that people tend to talk about the tendency for the body to droop or sag downward when they reach their 30th or 40th birthday. One authority stated that if all Americans were to lose fat and reach an optimal level of body composition, the energy in the fat could supply the annual residential electrical power needed in a group of cities including Boston, Chicago, San Francisco, and Washington, DC. Americans are not only wasting a lot of energy but they are doing so at the expense and damage of their own bodies and psyches.

Disadvantages of Obesity

A number of medical and health problems are related to excess fatness. If you are looking for several reasons to shed some pounds and optimize your body composition consider the following. As mentioned earlier, type 2 diabetics (noninsulin-dependent) do produce insulin; as a matter of fact, they tend to produce more insulin than nondiabetics. The condition involves a decreased number and/or function of insulin receptors lining the cells of the body. Therefore, although the insulin is present in the blood, it does not attach as easily to the lining of the cells and so glucose or blood sugar does not move into the cells as readily.

Two factors affect these insulin receptors: the amount of fat tissue and the degree of physical activity. More fat and less physical activity impair the receptors, thus making one prone to noninsulin-dependent diabetes. However, unlike insulin-dependent diabetes, a reduction of body fat and an increase in physical activity improve the function of the insulin receptors so that glucose can penetrate the cells and be used as an energy source. To a large extent type 2 diabetes may be preventable as well as reversible. These are important findings because about 90% of all diabetics are this particular type. Because susceptibility to the condition seems to be a genetic trait, maintenance of a relatively lean, physically active body is fundamental to prevention, particularly if type 2 diabetes exists in the family.

Other physical disadvantages of obesity include increased risk of heart disease, high blood pressure, varicose veins, hemorrhoids, hiatal hernia, arthritis, gout, low backache, and cancer.

A number of studies also indicate that obese people have lower ratings of self-concept. This observation probably indicates that no one wants to be much overweight: We don't feel as good, don't have as much energy and are therefore not as productive, and don't look as good as we might. A low self-concept undoubtedly limits a person in many ways because it alters the perception of how you relate to the rest of the world. The noteworthy thing to remember here, however, is the potentially great effect that can occur if the self-concept can be raised. If weight can be normalized and thus contribute to self-concept, the likelihood of additional changes being made is greatly enhanced. This may explain a common observation in people who begin exercise programs. As they modify their physical being, they often alter eating and smoking habits, become interested in stress management, and so on. In short, they become interested in other ways of improving themselves, which is a reflection of their self-concept. A healthy self-concept seems to increase the likelihood of good health habits overall.

Being overweight makes simple physical tasks more laborious, making a person less likely to be very physical. The irony is that moderate obesity encourages a reduction in physical activity, which over time decreases total fitness. Physical work and exercise become increasingly less attractive. With continued decline of physical activity, a person loses muscle mass and the metabolic rate slows. Now fewer calories are needed to fuel the body but eating habits typically remain the same. These changes occur gradually, and finally people may be shocked as they closely analyze their figures in a mirror. For such people, lack of energy is one of the most common complaints. It shouldn't be surprising to find that one of the most common psychological changes reported in polls and surveys regarding why people exercise is an increased mental and physical vigor.

Societal Standards

Although the purpose of this chapter is to aid people, particularly diabetics, to safely lose fat and to permanently stay healthily lean, I preface any remarks regarding how to do this by first discussing the standards of today's society regarding being slim. While the "trim is in" standard has created the desire by many people to be lean and fit, which is primarily very desirable, I think many people have false notions as to how far or to what extent they can actually change their body shape. The Miss America "36-24-36" physique is one that is produced mostly from heredity rather than exercise or diet. People in sports medicine use the term somatotype to describe the variety of body shapes which exist. From years of research with athletes and people training with weights, running, and other physical activities, we realize that the magnitude of change associated with training and diet can proceed only so far. If you were born with broad shoulders and hips, and thick wrists and ankles, you are going to look "squat" or broad no matter how slim you might become. In addition, if your limbs are short in proportion to your height, you will appear even broader. To a fullback or tackle on the football team, this may pose no hindrance. Actually, it may be an advantage in terms of lifting heavy weights or minimizing injury in contact sports. Also, in men such a physique lends itself to appearing muscular. Many boys and men would love to possess such a body build. However, a female with the same physical traits wishing to mimic today's TV and movie stars is forever doomed to failure if she tries to reshape her figure to the extent of looking like her idols. All the dieting, exercise, and willpower in the world won't change her bone structure. I've often told students, "You can't make a plow horse into a quarter horse."

So, I urge you, no, I beseech you, to set a reasonable goal for yourself. Don't exaggerate the importance of what you look like. It is a cultural flaw that we use the slim model with an ectomorphic physique to sell soft drinks, clothing, food, cars, and a thousand other products. Madison Avenue and Hollywood have proclaimed that the small percentage of women born to a bony configuration akin to Bo Derek and Linda Evans should reign supreme! Women of the world, you vast majority in the middle of the bell-shaped normal curve, you should arise to proclaim that women of all shapes and sizes can be beautiful, healthy, and yes, even sexy. But please, do not force yourself into someone else's idea of femininity.

What of the lean ladies who tend to great proficiency as joggers, hikers, and cross-country skiers? Many of you wish to add pounds but like your sisters with breadth and width, you too will change only so far with diet or training. Exercise of the resistance or strength type will promote a moderate increase in muscle mass, which will bring you closer to the mean, but most will never reach the "36-24-36" goal.

I emphasize my attention to females first because women have to bear the brunt of a male society's image regarding what women should look like. However, boys and men have pressure cast on them too. Call it the macho image, the John Wayne image, or whatever, but our culture ascribes the following physical traits as masculine: broad shoulders, narrow hips and fairly tall. Again, as in the case with women, few men are born with a bone structure with all these traits. Even with extensive weight training, few men would ever be a reasonable facsimile of Mr. America, although they may be able to make a greater change in contour than females because they can add significantly more muscle mass to their frames with training. However, the lean, ectomorphic distance runner types seem less able to gain muscle mass with resistance training probably because more of their muscle cells are the smaller, endurance type (slow-twitch cells) rather than the thicker, stronger type (fast-twitch cells). Also, a man with long extremities who gains some muscle will not appear to have increased in muscle mass as much as a man with short extremities. Typically men who are furthest from the muscular mesomorphic body type will be least able to dramatically change their body type with training.

If strength training is still unable to develop the "ideal" male or female body build, the only other approach lean, long men and women can employ is to overeat and gain more body fat. In terms of health, this approach is ridiculous, yet I've heard many young males say that they are eating more food to gain more size. Such statements are particularly true of young athletes. Unfortunately, you can't eat your way to greater muscularity. Eating excessively to gain bulk for whatever reason is simply unhealthy.

As a last point, let me remind you that the concept of beauty seems to change. To the ancient Athenian, the most pleasing male physique was one that depicted the capacity to do many things well. They probably would abhor today's body builder. From the great works of art produced during the Renaissance it is obvious that female beauty was characterized by considerably more bulk and plumpness than today. In short, during the Renaissance probably many more women possessed a figure that their culture deemed as pleasing. No one knows what physical traits society will value in the years ahead. In the meantime, be realistic. Our culture should promote a philosophy of being more concerned with health and function and less concerned with what we look like. We should judge others by what they do and not by their appearance. Judge yourself the same way.

Women and Weight Control

Women often note that they eat more before their menstrual periods. A recent study examined the daily basal metabolic rate of women and observed that it increased markedly 7 to 10 days prior to the onset of menstruation. The difference in energy expenditure between this phase of the cycle and the least active metabolic phase totalled about 350 calories per day, which was closely related to the 500 calorie variance in food intake at these times.

Women also find that weight loss becomes more difficult once they enter menopause. As the secretion of estrogen decreases at this time of life, women are more limited in removing fat from its storage sites. Women also retain fluid prior to their periods, which increases their body weight a bit. Thus, the variation in women's sex hormone secretion seems to make weight loss more variable for women than for men as well as more difficult. What is more, women typically have more fat and less muscle than men, resulting in a metabolic rate about 6% to 7% lower. For all of these reasons, women are not able to lose fat as easily as men. Recognition of this difference may encourage females to take a realistic approach in their plan to control weight. These sex differences in the ability to lose fat make it appear that men are more disciplined in dieting than women. There are no data to support this. Avoid the comparison with men regarding fat loss because it isn't a fair one.

The average woman's physique is more endomorphic or rounder and fuller than a man's. The woman's shorter legs, lower center of gravity and wider pelvis make her appear rounder. Remember that diet and exercise will not remove the primary bony configuration of your skeleton.

Do We Even Need Fat in Our Bodies?

For all the negative things we hear about excess weight, one might think an absence of fat might provide optimal health. However, several vital biological functions are fulfilled by fat. For example, some fat is needed to cushion the vital organs; the membrane of every living cell is partly comprised of fat; and vitamins A, D, E, and K are stored in fatty tissues. Experts believe a certain minimum of total body weight should be fat. This minimum is termed essential fat because it is needed to provide the functions listed. In adult men and women, this amount is estimated to be about 3% and 13% of the total body weight, respectively. Consequently, having less fat than this may jeopardize health.

How Much Fat Is too Much?

To answer this question adequately, realize that the criterion for fatness or obesity is not body weight alone but the ratio of fat weight to total body weight. Height-weight tables do not measure the former and so are of limited use. As a matter of fact, height-weight tables may be very misleading. Using the tables, a 6-foot 3-inch 220-pound football player with magnificent muscularity might be judged overweight while a plump, soft 180-pound sedentary college student of the same height might be termed "normal." The reverse could well be true. That is, many large muscular athletes have relatively low fat percentages as measured by the underwater weighing technique while some sedentary people with small bone structure have surprisingly high percentages of fat. I imagine many people hopping off a scale with the height-weight and frame size data affixed to the scale select their frame size after they have weighed themselves. Thus, you can always select a large frame and let the rating "normalize" according to the frame size you select.

A second misleading way to judge body fat is by comparison with weight at some previous occasion such as graduation from high school or college. That seems silly as it doesn't take into account what the body composition was at that earlier time. If one was too fat then, does that justify being as fat today? This comparison becomes even more invalid when it is realized that as we age, we tend to lose lean tissue such as bone and muscle while we tend to gain fat tissue. So, even if you weighed the same at high school as you did at age 40 or 50, you would not expect that weight to be composed of the same amount of muscle, fat or bone. A photograph of yourself some years ago and a view into a full-length mirror would probably support this statement.

The only valid widely available means of assessing body composition is measurement of fat in the skin using an instrument called a skinfold caliper. The procedure is only as good, however, as the skills of the tester and the quality of the caliper. Consequently, I suggest contacting the physical education department of a university or college near you to perform this test. They will have trained personnel as well as good instruments to accurately do this. Some departments will even have a special tank for weighing people underwater in their exercise physiology laboratory. For a reasonable fee you could probably take either of these tests. The underwater weighing procedure has the advantage of being more accurate. Using either of the tests described, the results greatly aid deciding how much weight should be lost.

Although no universal acceptance has been reached about specific levels of percent body fat, experts in sports medicine seem to agree that the fat composition in men should not exceed 20% to 25% while for women it should not exceed 30% to 35%. Beyond these levels, various disease states previously described occur in much greater frequency. Again, let me reemphasize that becoming excessively lean is not related to better health and in many sports it is not consistently related to better performance. Current data indicate that thousands of young females are anorexic or bulimic. Whether one rejects eating or forces oneself to vomit after binge-eating, both states should be recognized as psychological abnormalities. Women should also realize that rapid and excessive weight loss disrupts the normal menstrual cycle.

What Causes Obesity?

While it used to be popular for overweight people to claim that a glandular disorder such as an underactive thyroid caused their obesity, current medical data show that such disorders only explain about 1 out of every 1100 cases of obesity. There may be, however, a genetic component in obesity. In families where neither parent is obese, only about 14% of the children are found to be obese. About 40% to 50% of children in families with one parent overweight are also overweight; when both parents are overweight, the incidence rises to 75% to 80%.

There is also a positive relationship in the fatness of siblings; that is, lean children tend to have lean brothers and sisters, while obese children tend to have obese brothers and sisters. It is well known that animals can be bred to be larger and fatter while no change in diet is made. With humans, however, it is difficult to sort out environmental factors. While breeding experiments in humans cannot be done, data on twins and adopted children allow some interesting comparisons to be made. The results of such studies, however, tend to be inconclusive. A relationship has been found in some studies between adopted children and the biological parent as well as between twins, while no relationships have been observed in other studies. Based on the results of animal studies, however, several authorities conclude that heredity is a component in human obesity and that when obesity is well established or long lasting, it is very resistant to change.

Some research evidence indicates that exercise has little effect in extreme obesity. Rats placed on high fat diets early in life were found to have greatly increased appetites during youth and adulthood. Furthermore, the high fat diet accelerated weight gain even though caloric intake was normal. Most surprising of all, even the offspring of these animals were obese and had increased appetites. Part of the explanation for the potent weight-gaining effect of fat is that the body uses and stores fat more efficiently than carbohydrate and protein. Obesity is not a world-wide problem but appears only in cultures such as the United States where dietary fat intake is high. If these results of animal research can be applied to humans, then even exercise and dietary modification may be of limited value in the extremely obese. However, as with many disease states, prevention seems far more effective than cure. A change in the American diet to significantly reduce fat intake is suggested by such studies.

One of the most puzzling facets of obesity is the consistent observation that some people gain little or no weight when they overeat while others gain considerable weight, although no difference in physical activity exists. It appears most people have a mechanism to burn extra calories that doesn't seem to exist in the obese. Consequently, most people hold a fairly constant body weight and adapt metabolically to variations in caloric intake. A number of studies suggest that the mechanism involved is a special variety of fat tissue called brown fat. It differs from the more common yellow or white fat because it contains an abundance of structures called mitochondria, which also provide the dark color. Mitochondria are the sites in the cells where chemical reactions involving oxygen occur. The special function of brown fat is believed to be heat production. Animals that hibernate and animals exposed to cold weather have more brown fat, which keeps them warm. Possession of many mitochondria is analogous to possessing an extra metabolic furnace in the body. This fat appears in special locations of the body such as the back of the neck and backbone, which has allowed researchers to probe the fat to measure its temperature. As one would expect, brown fat is warmer than yellow fat.

Rats genetically disposed to obesity have difficulty adjusting to cold because their brown fat fails to increase its metabolic activity. In one study, when rats were placed on a human "junk food diet" containing 80% more calories than normal, they gained weight but the gain was only 27% of the initial weight. As they gained weight consuming this diet, total body energy expenditure increased. The increased metabolism appeared to be due almost entirely to increased metabolic activity in the brown fat. The temperature of the brown fat rose significantly.

Brown fat temperature is increased due to stimulation by the sympathetic nervous system. When one of the nerve transmitter substances at the sympathetic nerve endings (norepinephrine) is administered to humans, the temperature of brown fat increases. In obese women, brown fat activity is not increased as much as in nonobese women when this substance is administered. So, obese people may have a defect in their ability to increase the activity of their brown fat, which in turn may limit their ability to perk up the metabolism when excess calories are consumed. Secondly, autopsies reveal that some people possess no brown fat. The amount of brown fat one possesses can be increased by eating five or six meals per day instead of the standard three. Also, because norepinephrine is secreted during exercise, consistent physical activity stimulates brown fat development.

The Role of Exercise in Weight Control

To appreciate the role of exercise in weight control, some background information is needed. As a result of considerable research, many experts now believe that the single most common cause of obesity is lack of physical activity. Support for this contention includes the following observations: Obesity is nearly unknown in Third World nations where considerable daily physical activity is common; in temperate climates people typically gain several pounds of weight in the cold months of the year when they spend less time outside; sedentary people performing aerobic exercise lose weight although they usually gain several pounds of muscle simultaneously; we eat fewer calories today than in 1900 but are heavier and fatter; people who exercise aerobically eat more but are lighter and leaner. You may find it motivating to realize you can lose weight without having to semistarve yourself. As a matter of fact, once you optimize your weight and if you burn several hundred calories in exercise daily, you will more than likely be able to eat more than you do now and yet maintain the leanness you developed. Studies of Olympic marathon runners indicate they consume about 6,000 to 8,000 calories daily. That's a lot of food! Philippine sugar cane cutters who hack with a machete for hours at a time consume about 5,000 calories daily. What's more, these men only weigh about 130 pounds.

Excess body fat enhances not only the maintenance of fat put on but actually encourages the storage of more fat. When we gain weight, fat cells enlarge to store more fat. In one study, prisoners purposely overate to gain weight. Most of them experienced endocrine and metabolic changes. Insulin production increased, which not only raised their appetites but also enhanced the deposit of fat in their adipose tissue. Many studies also show that when weight is lost people become more physically active. Obesity breeds inactivity because it makes most physical activity harder to do, more awkward, less efficient, and certainly less enjoyable. So, once you gain weight, a vicious cycle becomes established that has the effect of making it difficult to lose weight. There is hope, however, as you will see.

What I've found so helpful as a diabetic is that I'm able to eat a good number of calories each day and yet I am able to stay lean, healthy, and fit. I'm even able to splurge on occasion without suffering a rise in blood sugar as a result of expending an unusually large amount of energy.

Exercise Prescription for Weight Control

The two major factors in designing an exercise program to lose fat and then to keep it off are the expenditure of a significant number of calories and the development and maintenance of muscle mass. A number of studies have made it clear that for exercise by itself to cause fat loss in adults, about

300 to 400 calories must be expended three or more times weekly. This may seem like a large number of calories but it may surprise you to know just how many calories are burned in various types of exercise. First of all, the key to energy expenditure is selection of a fairly vigorous intensity that can be sustained for 30 or more minutes. The more fit you are, the greater the intensity of exercise you can maintain for 30 minutes. For example, a fit person may be able to burn 15 or more calories each minute of aerobic exercise while a novice exerciser may only be able to sustain a vigor of exercise equivalent to 7 or 8 calories each minute. In 30 minutes of exercise at these given intensities, the fit subject would expend 450 calories while the novice would burn about half that number. For this reason, less fit people typically have to exercise for more than 30 minutes to reach the threshold level of 300 calories. Fairly fit people will typically burn 300 plus calories in 30 minutes. As previously stated, you cannot safely start an exercise program exercising for such long periods. This would assuredly invite a variety of possible overuse injuries leading to a visit with an orthopedist. So, realize that it will take several weeks before you will be able to exercise long enough and vigorously enough to expend 300 calories. However, to minimize injury as well as to make exercise more enjoyable, I favor activity emphasizing duration rather than intensity. Because blood vessel blockage is present to some extent in most adults, particularly men, lower intensity exercise is far safer.

Another reason for not overemphasizing high intensity exercise to aid in weight loss is because a greater production of lactic acid occurs. Lactic acid inhibits the release of fat from deposit sites throughout the body. Consequently, the active muscles in high intensity exercise burn more carbohydrate and less fat each minute. The utilization of fat as an energy source during exercise is maximized by emphasizing duration with intensity at or below 50% of maximum. This 50% of maximum work capacity is also considered to be the lowest level of work that elicits a cardiorespiratory training effect. So, although the 50% of maximum intensity is not particularly vigorous work, it will provide a conditioning effect as well as allow a good number of calories to be expended for people starting an exercise program.

To integrate what has been discussed up to this point, Table 8 summarizes an aerobic program for a hypothetical sedentary 50-year-old with no medical problems. The program is designed to provide an aerobic training effect but also to facilitate fat loss. Note that a 5-minute warm-up and 5-minute cool-down are performed as a regular part of each session. I am estimating that 25 calories are expended in each of these periods. I have selected 15 minutes as the initial duration to minimize injuries. The duration of each exercise session is increased every 2 weeks by 5 minutes, a conservative increment meant to protect the participant from overuse injury. Assuming that the subject's maximum aerobic capacity or maximum oxygen uptake is 3 liters, a typical value for an average size 50-year-old sedentary male, exercise at 50% of this value is equivalent to 7.5 calories each minute. By the fifth week, note that the calories expended each minute have increased to nine. This moderate increase in energy expenditure per minute is typical because as you become better-trained aerobically, the maximum oxygen uptake increases as does the percent of maximum that can be comfortably tolerated. This second training change may largely reflect a greater anaerobic threshold, which is the workload where lactic acid accumulates faster than it can be dissipated. As the weeks of training go by, people usually increase the speed of walking, swimming, cycling, and other activities because of these reasons, and they do so voluntarily and probably unconsciously because they are simply capable of working more briskly although their perception of this new work effort remains unchanged. Although moving faster and burning more energy, the training heart rate may still be about the same since the person is now able to consume more oxygen and burn more energy per minute at the same heart rate. This occurs because the heart ejects more blood per beat or contraction and so does not have to beat faster.

The training heart rate equivalent to 50% of maximum aerobic capacity is about 60% to 65% of maximum. Because of the explanation given in the previous paragraph, you do

Table 8   Starter Aerobic Exercise Program for Weight Loss for a Person Weighing 150 Pounds

Week	Duration (minutes)	Intensity[1]	Estimated calories expended per minute	Estimated calories expended per session[2]
1 and 2	15	50% of maximum aerobic capacity or about 65% of maximum HR	7.5	162.5
3 and 4	20		7.5	180
5 and 6	25		9.0	275
7 and 8	30		9.0	320
9 and 10	35		11.0	435
11 and 12	40		11.0	490

[1]Intensity is the same through the 12 weeks.
[2]Includes the energy expended in a 5-minute warm-up and 5-minute cool-down.

not necessarily have to increase the training heart rate if the primary goal is weight reduction. My experience, however, indicates that people gradually increase intensity over the first several months of training. If a person performed the routine prescribed in Table 8 three days weekly, by the seventh week more than 300 calories would be expended each session. The subject has likely reached the 300-calorie weight loss threshold with a minimum chance of injury due to the gradual progression and inclusion of a warm-up and cool-down. Once this level has been reached, the subject could leave all components the same and enter a maintenance phase of exercise. The passage of several more months of exercise would result in continued loss of body fat, however. If the intensity was increased slightly, say to 12 calories per minute, then 530 calories would be expended per session. One could easily get carried away and begin to think of the large number of calories burned in sessions lasting more than an hour. However, because the injury rate rises markedly when activity goes much beyond 30 minutes, let me urge you to limit yourself to 30 to 40 minutes. I think a better strategy than increasing exercise duration beyond 40 minutes is to exercise four or five times weekly rather than just three times. Whereas three 40-minute weekly sessions at 11 calories per minute result in nearly 1,500 calories burned per week, four sessions result in nearly 2,000 and five sessions would allow an expenditure of nearly 2,500 calories.

To minimize the likelihood of injury to someone who wishes to exercise more than three times weekly, there is a decided value in selecting alternative forms of exercise. If you normally walk, then you can cycle, swim, or cross-country ski on the extra days, which will allow you to burn added calories and have some fun with a different activity.

Because a pound of fat is equivalent to about 3,500 calories, we can now determine about how long it will take to lose a specific amount of fat. Using the data already given, that is, 490-calorie workouts performed three times a week, in weeks 11 and 12 you would expend 1,470 calories. At this level of exercise it would take 2.4 weeks to lose 1 pound of fat. While this seems like a very slow way to lose weight, realize that this weight is lost with no change whatsoever in diet. Secondly, the weight lost is mostly fat tissue and not water and protein as is the case with the majority of weight lost in quick weight loss schemes. One key principle in weight loss is that the loss of fat cannot be accomplished in a short time. When most people lose weight rapidly it is mostly water. Therefore they regain the weight (i.e., water) very quickly. As we all know, it's easy to lose weight but hard to keep it off. *The physiology of fat loss requires a long-term change in habits so that the loss is gradual and mostly fat.* You may want to underline the previous sentence and refer to it often in the next several months. These hard, cold facts may help sustain your motivation.

A later section in this chapter deals with the nutritional and dietary facets of weight control. For now, let me just add that fat loss will be accelerated if a moderate reduction in calorie intake accompanies the onset of your exercise program. A daily reduction of 500 calories will sum to a net deficit of

3,500 calories in just 1 week. If you reduced food intake by 500 calories daily and expended 500 calories daily in exercise, then the total daily caloric deficit is 1,000 calories. At this rate, one could lose 1 pound of fat every 3 1/2 days. A range of numbers you should memorize is the maximum weight loss per week: 1 or 2 pounds. This recommended maximum has been accepted by professional nutritionists and the American Medical Association because research indicates that weight loss beyond this rate is largely due to the loss of water and the breakdown of protein. These are unhealthy changes and if carried to an extreme can actually lead to death. Remember the rule about weight loss: To be safe it must be slow and gradual.

The second ingredient in an effective exercise program for weight control deals with maintenance of an elevated metabolism. Metabolism represents the amount of energy used to accomplish a specific activity. Basal metabolism is the energy used at complete rest. The energy released could be measured in terms of heat production or oxygen consumed by the entire body. While many factors affect metabolism, two that deal with exercise are discussed here. One key factor is the amount of muscle mass in the entire body. All other things being equal, a more muscular person will require more calories than will a less muscular person even if the total body weights are identical. That's hardly surprising. I am not advocating that you need to train like a body builder to significantly increase your metabolism. A little bit of strength-type exercise will do a lot in terms of adding to or maintaining your muscle mass.

The resting or basal metabolism typically decreases about 3% each decade after the age of 25 to 30 years. This is not so much an age threshold as much as it is a loss of muscle mass threshold. At age 37 or 38, the average person needs about 3% fewer calories than he or she did at age 25 to 30; in the late 40s, the difference is about 6%, and so on. Because we know that muscle strength and mass can be maintained reasonably well with only two training sessions per week, it holds that two weekly sessions of appropriate weight training or body resistance exercises will be effective in maintaining a higher metabolic rate. As discussed in the chapter on muscular fitness, a selection of exercises that work many muscles simultaneously is an efficient means of stimulating many muscles in a short workout. One pushing, one pulling, one leg, and one abdominal exercise can be performed in about 10 minutes. Spending 20 minutes a week to keep your muscles functional and your metabolism up is well worth the time.

The second exercise factor affecting the overall body metabolism is the extra energy expended after exercise. For decades, exercise physiologists have measured the oxygen or energy consumed during various types of sport and work. Data are available in many books and articles specifying the calories expended in such activities. Only recently, however, have we realized that metabolism remains elevated for several hours after a typical exercise session. The longer and more intense the exercise, the greater and longer the elevation is. It is difficult at present to specify the number of extra calories expended in the recovery hours after exercise, but we can at least take comfort in knowing that we burn considerably more calories than the values indicated in most books and articles in print today. It has been estimated that a person might lose about 5 pounds in a year purely due to this elevation in metabolism in the recovery period after exercise. One study found that metabolism was increased 12% for each degree of body temperature (centigrade) raised. It is largely the rise in body temperature that seems to keep metabolism increased after exercise.

Isn't There Any Easier Way? What About Saunas, Body Wraps, and Vibration Devices?

These techniques fall within the category of quackery. As the saying goes, "There's a sucker born every minute." Saunas and steam rooms do cause one to sweat but the weight loss involved is only temporary and is only water rather than fat. Using the best of my imagination I am unable to think of even a halfway credible explanation as to how body wraps could work. The explanations one reads in the back pages of magazines are quite comical yet thousands of people spend money hoping for a magic cure. What optimists we are. Some advertisements propose that vibration belts and rollers jiggle the fat causing it to break down. Some have even said it specifically eliminates cellulite. Cellulite is not a medical or scientific term but has been used by various pseudoexperts to describe the uneven, bumpy fat deposits some women have in the thighs. Some refer to it as the orange peel-looking fat.

As is probably known by most people, none of these techniques have any scientific merit. They simply do not work and they create false hopes that may keep people from using sound techniques. Furthermore, agencies such as the Food and Drug Administration are not able to keep up with such schemes.

Will Exercise Increase My Appetite?

This is a question people frequently ask. Implied in the question, I think, is the possibility that an increase in appetite will occur after exercise and lead to overeating. Interestingly, with moderate levels of energy expenditure in humans, about 100 to 400 calories, appetite is actually depressed by several hormones secreted during activity (for example, catecholamines and dopamine). The level of these hormones in the blood remains elevated for an hour or two following exercise. So, the appetite suppressant effect is not particularly long-lasting, but some suggest that if a meal is taken not long after a bout of exercise, less food will be eaten. This would seemingly be a realistic application of the physiology involved. Even a brisk walk before dinner would help in this regard as the same hormone release is produced even in light exercise.

On the low end of the activity spectrum, if a person or animal is deprived of physical activity (deprived seems a fitting word to me), the appetite is increased. Farmers have probably known this for a long time but researchers had to substantiate it experimentally with animals and humans. To pen or corral an animal and reduce grazing and movement to a minimum is all too similar to the sparseness of movement characteristic of much of our existence. We drive everywhere: to school, work, or shopping, even if the destination is a mere block or two away. Even the children are driven everywhere.

In the school system where we live, children are bused if they live more than a mile from the assigned school. Some children are even driven to the bus stop by their parents. Then our children sit for hours on end in school; they are lucky if they have a physical education class more than once or twice a week, and then they are driven home again. They recuperate at home by watching cable television or movies on the home VCR, or log some time on the home computer. It certainly is no wonder children today are fatter than even 10 or 20 years ago. Recently published test results involving thousands of school children indicate this. We adults, however, shouldn't shake our heads or fingers too vigorously because most of our day is just as sedentary. The data simply show that daily exercise has to be planned for our children as well as ourselves. A lot more of us could park a few blocks from work and walk for 5 or 10 minutes twice a day. It's a lot more persuasive to motivate children to walk to school if they realize that mom and dad also walk. Families should discuss fitness, obesity, and health and develop some guidelines. It may prompt some of the family members who are not regular exercisers to get started and develop an exercise habit.

The appetite is stimulated if more than about 400 calories are expended per day in work and sport. This explains the greater food and caloric intake of some of our serious running and exercise friends. It appears that the extra food consumed is primarily used to replenish the muscle fuel (glycogen) used during the physical activity. Otherwise, consecutive days of long, vigorous work would not be possible. There is also a point in exercise where even the appetite does not allow one to eat enough to fully compensate for the energy expended. For example, lean, well-trained mountain climbers typically lose 10 to 15 pounds during a climb lasting a week or more.

Two Secrets of Youth

Do you remember "having" to go home for dinner when you were a youngster? Being outside with your friends playing was so much fun, so inviting, that having to break away for a meal was actually viewed as a distraction and bother.

Most adults run to the dinner table all too eagerly; perhaps we perceive eating as too enjoyable. I think a tendency in our culture is to place too much emphasis on eating as a source of enjoyment and recreation. A local poll in Omaha, Nebraska, where I live, showed that dining out was the number one source of recreation. I enjoy eating and dining out, but I don't think it is my number one fun thing to do. I love to run, play basketball, read, and play ball with my children. I don't think eating is in my top five. I wonder if it is with children? What about you? Perhaps the message is people should concentrate on things besides eating.

A second "secret" many children seem to have learned is that after eating you do not sit down. Now that's a toughie for me, because my typical day includes relaxing immediately after dinner, reading the newspaper, and watching the news on TV. When I was 8, 10, 12, and 14 years old, however, after eating I was back on my feet immediately after a meal and physically active. My children seem to follow the same pattern. There appears to be some relationship between what we do after eating and how much fat we have. The researchers once again have observed and studied the pattern and sure enough, we burn a few more calories in doing the same physical tasks after having eaten as compared to doing them on an empty stomach. Kids are right! The digestion of food requires burning calories; our metabolism is increased above its basal or resting state by about 20% after eating. This is termed the thermic effect. When the meal is followed by exercise there is a doubling of the thermic effect. Thus, exercise after eating reduces the calories you would otherwise store as fat but the exercise also burns calories in itself.

A helpful pattern to use in weight control would be to exercise moderately for even 5 to 10 minutes after each meal. Since we diabetics tend to have an elevation in blood sugar in the first hour or two following eating, how effective it would be to follow some of our meals, particularly dinner because it is usually the largest, with some light exercise. I find this quite easy to do in the spring, summer and early fall when the weather is nice. I feel my evening blood sugar is better controlled this way. I often walk, play ball, bicycle, or cut the grass after eating dinner. Typically it is an activity that is rather low intensity. I don't think my stomach would appreciate vigorous exercise immediately after eating. Researchers have found that a feeding of less than 500 calories, provided it is mostly carbohydrate, does not even detract from all-out performance such as running a 1-mile race. Note that children usually eat small meals but snack in between. They seem to have figured this out.

Try incorporating some of these "secrets of youth" into your life. I think more value may be associated with them than meets the eye.

How Many Sit-ups and Trunk Twisters Will It Take to Reduce My Waist?

I caught you, didn't I? I did if you were looking for an answer with a number in it. However, exercise will not reduce fat at specific sites. In other words, although sit-ups or trunk curls will strengthen the abdominal muscles, they will not thin the layer of fat in the skin overlying these muscles. To reduce fat in the abdominal region or hips or anywhere else, more energy must be expended than consumed for a period of weeks or months. This is why aerobic activities that burn so many calories are so beneficial in weight loss.

If I Develop My Muscles With Exercise, Won't They Turn Into Fat Once I Stop Exercising?

No, they will not because muscle cells cannot be converted into fat cells, kidney cells, epithelial cells, or any other kind of cell. The source of this misconception stems from the observation that after a muscular person stops training, the musculature is reduced in size and strength or is said to be atrophied. If the person continues eating the same number of calories while the muscles are shrinking in size, more fat accumulates in the skin. Our once lean and strong friend is now less muscular and more fat. His body composition has changed and since the two types of tissue changed gradually at the same time, it may appear to an observer that the muscles turned into fat.

Influence of Exercise on Nutritional Status

Many studies have shown that physically active people are not only leaner than sedentary people but they also consume more food. A study comparing joggers with inactive people showed that the male joggers consumed 2,960 calories per day versus 2,360 for the inactive men; the women runners consumed 2,390 calories, while the inactive women consumed 1,820 calories. The absolute difference in each case is about 600 calories, a substantial difference. Per unit of body weight the difference is even greater. That is, the joggers consumed more calories per pound of body weight because they were lighter. One likely fringe benefit of this increased food intake on an absolute or relative basis is enhanced nutritional status. Dietary surveys of Americans of all ages indicate several nutrients including calcium, iron, magnesium, one or more of the B complex vitamins, and vitamin A are likely to be lacking in many individuals. An increased consumption of grains and dairy products would likely eliminate these deficiencies. By being physically active we cannot only afford the enjoyment of eating more but also are more likely to meet optimal nutritional standards.

Summary

It is obvious that exercise plays a major role in weight control. A summary of these effects may serve now and later as motivating evidence to stay physically active.

1.   Exercise of the proper type, frequency, intensity, and duration expends a large number of calories.
2.   A considerable number of calories are expended in the hours after exercise primarily because the body temperature and metabolic rate remain elevated.
3.   Exercise helps curb the appetite by reducing insulin secre-

tion (except in type 1 diabetics) and by releasing several hormones (catecholamines and dopamine).

4. Strength-type exercise helps to maintain muscle mass, which in turn keeps the basal metabolic rate relatively high. Thus, even at rest a person with good muscular development expends more calories than a person with lesser muscular development.

5. Endurance exercise increases the production of brown fat, which elevates the metabolic rate.

6. Endurance training enhances the ability to take fat from the storage sites and use it as an energy source within the muscles during exercise. Therefore, more fat and less carbohydrate is burned per minute of endurance exercise when the muscles are endurance trained.

7. The speed with which food passes through the small and large intestine is greater in fit people. Consequently, fewer calories are absorbed after digestion.

8. More calories are burned in exercise when performed soon after eating as compared to doing the same exercise on an empty stomach.

9. Because fit, active people expend more calories and have an increased metabolic rate, they typically need more food and therefore, eat more food. One advantage of this is an improved nutritional status.

Lastly, exercise has strong potential to add fun and enjoyment to your life while dietary restriction represents a negative factor, a taking away or deprivation. I think it is likely that exercise can become part of anyone's lifestyle because exercise can be fun, fulfilling, and enhance the ego. Dietary changes, on the other hand, don't offer these benefits, and therefore dietary changes may be more difficult to instill in our habits.

Dietary Aspects of Weight Control

The influence of diet on human health has received great attention recently. Diet has been found to be related to obesity, cardiovascular disease, cancer, high blood pressure, and type 2 diabetes. The relationship between diet and weight control will be discussed in the remainder of this chapter.

Fad Diets and Rapid Weight Loss Techniques

The never ending development of new diets is fascinating to behold. Each month new regimens appear in women's magazines promising to take off pounds quickly. The before and after picture, the inclusion of a few scientific or medical terms, and a slightly incomplete explanation as to how the diet actually works seem to be common components in advertisements of these diets. To impress the reader and to hit us emotionally, the names of a few athletes or Hollywood personalities are mentioned. "Sylvia Superstar was once overweight, introverted, and unwanted. The XQ!R2K Diet, however, ____." You can fill in the blanks as well as I can.

The pseudodiets also often have a proper noun in the title, such as the Stillman Diet, Cambridge Diet or Scarsdale Diet. The association with a name perhaps is intended to make the diet seem credible or official. Some of the recent fad diets are based on special substances such as eggs and grapefruit, alcohol (remember this one?), liquid amino acids, protein powder, vinegar-kelp-cider, algae, glucomannan, and starch blockers. However, if they were all so marvelous, why do new substances and regimens continually replace the old? Alcohol, for example, is not only high in calories (7 calories per gram as compared to 4 per gram for carbohydrates) but it also stimulates the appetite. The hucksterism will continue, though. For a few dollars, thousands of Americans will invest and hope that a miraculous cure is possible. I think that most people sense intuitively that these schemes will not work. The schemes appeal to people's basically positive nature, sense of hope, and emotions. Most of us realize deep down that there are no miraculous foods or plans to control body weight.

The Dangers of Low Calorie-High Protein Diets

Many diets presented in magazines allow a total of only 1,000 to 1,200 calories per day to be consumed. I find this hard to accept because it does not take variation in body size into account. Does it seem logical to ask a 280-pound football player to consume the same number of calories as a 50-year-old woman who weighs 110 pounds? A vital fact commonly disregarded in such diets is that nutrient requirements are in fact related to body size. The football player does need more protein and probably all other nutrients than a much smaller person. Consequently, I don't think a general numerical value can be deemed appropriate for most people. The caloric intake should in part reflect the size of the person.

First assessing the number of calories typically eaten each day makes more sense; this requires careful record keeping. Note all foods and beverages consumed for 4 days including one weekend day. This provision gives a more meaningful estimate than if only weekdays were analyzed. Next analyze the content of the calories. You can do this using the values in a nutrition book or to simplify the process, you can have a detailed nutritional analysis done professionally. There are several excellent computer software programs available with which to do this. Contact the health, physical education, recreation department, or home economics department of a local college or university to see what they charge for such an analysis.

With the nutritional analysis, decide where you can best afford to delete some calories. For example, what percentage of your daily calories come from fats? Reduction of fat intake is a good place to start because of the health risks associated with a high fat intake and because fat is higher in calories than any other food type. Rather than attempting to make a sudden dramatic change, consider dropping your daily intake of fats by about 300 calories. That represents a rather modest change in your eating habits, which most people can tolerate reasonably well. In about 12 days this slight dietary change could result in the loss of 1 pound of fat if the rest of the diet stayed the same. If this dietary change was combined with a minimum of 3 to 4 days of aerobic exercise with each session expending about 300 to 400 calories, the loss of fat will be further accelerated. Together, a moderate increase in activity coupled with a moderate reduction in calories represents the safest and most effective way to lose fat while minimizing the loss of muscle mass and other proteins (e.g., red blood cells, white blood cells, and enzymes). This finding is supported by published studies in medical and physiology journals and is worth noting.

When the caloric consumption is decreased by more than about 500 calories, a good portion of the weight lost consists of proteins and water. Worse yet, valuable minerals or electrolytes are lost with the water, a potential danger because this mineral shortage makes the heart irritable and prone to loss of its rhythmic contractions. Cases of fatal heart attacks exist that autopsies have indicated to be caused by low mineral content, so many of the fad diets that cause severe water and mineral loss are more dangerous than realized. The liquid amino acid diet, popular in the late 1970s, was advocated as a safe way to lose weight and supposedly was designed to avoid the wasting of muscle and loss of other proteins. Although the amino acid supplement was to be the only source of calories, the tendency to break down tissue proteins was supposedly to be replaced by the amino acid supplement. The actual content of the supplement was chemically analyzed and found to vary greatly from the composition stated on the label. Some of the claimed contents were totally absent, whereas others were four times higher than stated. For whatever reasons, medical authorities attributed nearly 60 deaths to use of the supplement and diet. The cause of death in the majority of cases was heart irregularities related to inadequate mineral intake; none of the individuals had severe blockage of the coronary arteries.

As previously discussed, a key role of carbohydrates in our diet is to spare excessive breakdown of protein. If carbohydrate intake is limited, protein is converted into its building blocks of amino acids, which are then used to build glucose in the liver. One study demonstrated that a protein-supplemented fasting diet reduced the amount of certain proteins in the blood. One function of blood proteins is to maintain the volume of water in the blood. It does this in a process known as osmosis. When the blood protein level decreases, some water in the blood moves to surrounding tissues. If the blood protein level remains low, enough fluid can accumulate in some tissues to cause swelling or edema. The point is that extreme alterations of diet tend to promote problems and secondly, they are not effective in maintaining fat loss.

Recently, medical authorities have stated that people who frequently alter their diets dramatically in attempting to lose weight suffer irreparable damage. Elevation of blood pressure tends to be a by-product as does a decrease in metabolic rate. The metabolic rate apparently decreases because every time a person diets and significantly reduces the caloric intake, muscle tissue is lost. Once off the diet, the metabolic rate is lower due to the loss of muscle. Thereafter, the number of calories needed to maintain body weight and musculature is decreased. However, if eating habits return to the previous level, the extra calories are stored as fat. This negative cycle eventuates in a spiral of continually less muscle and a progressive lowering of the metabolic rate. This probably explains much of the reason why those who diet repeatedly are actually worse off than those who make no attempt at all. It doesn't really seem fair, but it is a fact that should be emphasized to those wishing to lose weight intelligently. These findings suggest that moderate changes in eating, such as the 300-calorie deficit recommended here, are not only safer medically speaking but also more effective and easier to accept psychologically.

Why Do the Fad Diets Cause a Faster Weight Loss Than the Safer Recommended Diets?

I pose this question to emphasize the dangers of quick loss schemes as well as their ineffectiveness. Normally, the body's total energy is supplied mostly by fat and carbohydrate. Protein contributes only about 3% to 5% of our energy supply and this percentage is not significantly altered in nondiabetics even during exercise, unless the supply of carbohydrate in the active muscles (called glycogen) is nearly exhausted. This condition, however, only occurs in long endurance activities such as marathoning, hiking, and long-distance cycling and swimming. At such times, protein is exchanged between the liver and muscle where it provides energy for muscle contraction; the liver uses components of muscle protein to produce glucose, which is transported in the blood back to muscles that are low in glucose and glycogen. Whereas this accentuated breakdown of protein doesn't occur for some 2 to 4 hours of exercise in nondiabetics, the process begins at about 40 minutes after the start of exercise in diabetics.

When the dietary intake of carbohydrate is limited as would occur when fasting or using a high protein-low carbohydrate diet, protein is degraded in a larger quantity than normal. The end products of protein breakdown, ammonia and urea, are always being produced in small quantities and are eliminated in the urine. These substances have a diuretic effect; that is, they stimulate urination, which helps to remove the chemicals from the body. The typical balance between ammonia and urea production and elimination results in a fairly constant level of these chemicals in the body. The balance established exemplifies the process of homeostasis or chemical balance. However, when proteins are broken down in larger than normal quantities, the excess ammonia and urea can only be eliminated by an extra volume of urine excreted. However, water and electrolytes are both lost in larger than normal amounts. Dieters using a rapid weight loss technique, if only using scale weight as a determinant of dieting success, may think they have lost fat when in reality it is mostly protein and water, and precious little fat has been lost. Hence, rapid weight loss diets that limit the amount of carbohydrate ingested do cause substantial and rapid weight loss but only a small amount of the weight loss is fat.

A second reason why we lose body water when on the typical fad diet is that when carbohydrate intake is inadequate, the byproducts of fat metabolism, called ketones, are accentuated. Diabetics know this word well because when ketones accumulate faster than they are removed, they appear in the

urine. It is an emergency signal that insulin intake is insufficient. When fat breakdown is interfered with by a shortage
of carbohydrate intake and utilization, ketones can rise to the
danger level. The term ketosis is used to describe this state.
The condition can lead to coma, unconsciousness, and even
death when allowed to go unchecked. Diabetics in ketosis
sometimes must be hospitalized and given massive doses of
insulin and fluids to prevent catastrophe. However, note that
the body, specifically the kidneys, attempts to maintain
homeostasis or a balanced chemical state by producing large
quantities of urine to wash out excess ketones. To a lesser extent, even nondiabetics who fast or extremely limit the intake
of carbohydrate produce extra ketones, which stimulates considerable water loss. Once again the scale indicates you have
lost weight but it certainly doesn't indicate what was lost. The
results of rapid weight loss are therefore paradoxical: Weight
is rapidly lost but little of it is fat. These effects are summarized in Figure 9.

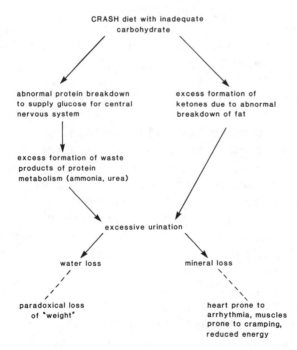

Figure 9 The physiology of rapid weight loss

The ability to change behavior in such a fundamental part of life as eating requires a certain level of maturity and honesty with yourself. The changes to be made are simple, but as is often the case, the simpler and more basic the act, the more difficult it is to change. The remainder of the chapter discusses how we can modify our eating habits to control weight and to obtain better balance of our blood sugar. All of the techniques and concepts are founded on published scientific research.

Carbohydrate Versus Fat

Although carbohydrates such as bread, pasta, and potatoes have typically been thought of as the first foods to be reduced or eliminated when trying to lose weight, they are not the caloric culprits people have supposed them to be. All carbohydrates, be they starch or sugar, contain about 4 calories per gram while fats contain about 9 calories per gram. Surprised? This fact is quite the opposite of what many of today's fad diets suggest. It is fats we should reduce in our diet, not carbohydrates. Two pats of butter or margarine equal 200 calories; 2 tablespoons of mayonnaise equal more than 200 calories; 2 tablespoons of cream in a cup of coffee yield 75 calories! We think of coffee as a zero calorie drink, but if you use 2 tablespoons of cream in each of four cups of coffee each day, that represents 300 calories. One could add a pound of fat to the body in about 12 days by switching from black coffee to coffee with cream. One could also lose a pound of fat by switching to black coffee, however. Diabetics in particular should realize that there are more than just a few calories in the cream added to coffee. The effects may not only be felt in your weight but also in your blood sugar. Such minor changes in diet do not demonstrate themselves by a quick weight gain. Rather, they tend to exert their effect slowly and insidiously.

Many groups including the American Heart Association and various groups of professional nutritionists have recommended that Americans should reduce their intake of total fat. Whereas the average American consumes about 40% to 43% of each day's calories from fat, it is recommended that fat should comprise only about 30% or less of the daily total energy supply. The rationale for this recommendation includes the high caloric value of fat but also the relationship of fat intake to cardiovascular disease and several types of cancer (e.g., colon and breast). It appears that an overly high intake of fat simply is not a good health habit.

A common misconception regarding fat is that a person only needs to watch the intake of margarine, butter, cream, and salad dressing to significantly reduce the ingestion of fat. A major source of dietary fat, however, comes from cakes, cookies, pastry, and meats. The touted high protein diets tend to be high fat diets and therefore high calorie diets. About 80% of the calories in lunchmeats such as bologna, salami, and hot dogs come from fat; a cup of shelled peanuts contains more than 800 calories! Potato chips, corn chips, and other salty, finger-food snacks tend to be high in calories because of their fat content. One cup of whole milk contains 160 calories while skim milk yields only about 90 calories. The caloric difference once again stems from the difference in fat content. The calories in 2% milk, by the way, are about midway between skim and whole milk. The 2% does not mean that 98% of the fat has been removed; actually less than half the fat is removed.

The way foods are prepared has a strong effect on their caloric and fat content. Frying foods is as common to American cuisine as is apple pie. (Pie crust is high in fat too.) The calories added to potatoes in making french fries, and the frying of chicken and fish convert relatively low-fat, low-calorie foods into caloric bombs. This is why eating out tends to be expensive calorically. If trying to lose weight and keep it off, you may be wise to limit eating out. Additionally, when eating in a restaurant, ask for the B items, that is, those that are baked, boiled, and broiled. Today's fitness-health emphasis has encouraged more and more restaurants to offer low calorie alternatives. Who ever thought McDonald's would have a salad bar? Today you can probably eat out more often and not pay the caloric price if you select restaurants that offer such foods and if you discipline yourself to make the appropriate choice most of the time.

The typical fast food meal is high in calories because of the relatively high fat content. A Burger King hamburger, french fries, and a milk shake yield about 1100 to 1200 calories. Similar foods at McDonald's and Arthur Treacher's provide about the same number of calories. For a diabetic, the intake of 1000 calories or more at one meal represents a potent mass of energy that will require a good deal of insulin if high blood sugar is to be avoided. The high fat nature of the food further adds to the burden of insulin. A high fat meal or diet, all other things being equal, requires more insulin than a meal of identical calories but of a different blend of food types.

Table 9 lists the percent of calories from fat and the total calories in various foods. Note that cheese, nuts, and meats are high in calories because they are high in fat. These foods should be limited in the diets of people trying to lose weight.

With the widespread availability and use of noncaloric or low-caloric sweeteners, it is interesting to note they do not seem to be effective in reducing the intake of calories. They do allow diabetics to consume "sweets" and perhaps satisfy a craving for them, but research indicates that people still eat

Table 9 Fat Content in Common Foods

Food	Calories per serving	% Calories from fat	Fat content in grams
Dairy products			
Whole milk, 1 cup	160	47	8
Ice cream, ¾ cup	143	48	11
Cheddar cheese, 2 oz	228	73	19
Swiss cheese, 2 oz	214	73	16
Cream cheese, 2 tbsp	99	88	10
Fish			
Salmon, sardines, herring, 4 oz	215	50	14
Tuna fish, canned in oil, 3 oz	170	31	7

(Cont.)

Table 9   (Cont.)

Food	Calories per serving	% Calories from fat	Fat content in grams
Meat (all visible fat trimmed)			
Chicken breast broiled, 3 oz	115	23	2
Club steak, 4 oz	277	48	15
Pork roast, 4 oz	287	50	16
Liverwurst, 2 oz	174	75	14
Hot dog, 2 oz	176	80	16
Bacon, 1 slice	45	80	5
Hamburger, regular, 3 oz	245	62	17
Veal cutlet, broiled, 3 oz	185	39	9
Nuts and seeds			
Peanut butter, 2 tbsp	188	73	16
Sunflower seeds, 1/8 cup	100	71	9
Almonds, 1/8 cup	123	77	11
Walnuts, 1/8 cup	98	79	9
Pastry			
Danish pastry	179	49	10
Apple pie	302	38	13
Miscellaneous			
Chocolate, 1 oz	147	53	9
Cream of mushroom soup, 10 oz	150	66	11
Fast foods			
McDonald's:			
Big Mac, fries and shake	1100	26	32
French fries	180	50	10
Chocolate shake	315	23	35
Pizza Hut:			
10-in supreme pizza	1200	26	35
Arthur Treacher's:			
3 pieces fish, chips, and slaw	1200	48	64
Kentucky Fried Chicken:			
3 pieces chicken, potatoes, roll, and slaw	1000	50	55
Arby's:			
Sliced beef sandwich, 2 potato patties, slaw, and shake	1200	30	40

as many calories by eating larger amounts of other foods. It's as though artificial sweeteners don't suppress our need for a basic number of calories, but they do permit the consumption of sweet-tasting foods and drinks without adding calories. I think what this country needs to help people lose weight is an artificial fat with no calories. How does Nutrafat sound?

Low Fat, Low Calorie Foods or How to Save 300 Calories a Day the Easy Way

The secret of making dietary changes or perhaps lifestyle changes of any type is to make them slowly and gradually. The savings of 300 calories each day adheres to this principle. The term diet implies a temporary change while the emphasis of this entire book is on permanent change. A reduction of only 300 calories will not leave you hungry at bedtime; the dietary changes suggested here may even make you feel more comfortably full after each meal than you otherwise would. An effective way to carve 300 calories from your daily diet is to reduce your fat intake. Table 10 shows a number of simple ways to do this.

The manner in which food is prepared is another factor that determines dietary intake of fat. Broiling, baking, and sautéing foods results in a large saving of calories as compared to frying. Also, by emphasizing foods high in carbohydrate you save calories. Only about 3% to 4% of the calories in beans and peas come from fat; most fruits have only a trace of fat; with the exception of such vegetables as avocados and olives, most vegetables also have only a trace of fat. Breads and oatmeal are about 12% fat, crackers 18%, doughnuts 43%, macaroni and spaghetti 5%, pancakes 30%, and dinner rolls 22% fat. It should be evident that a diet high in carbohydrates tends to be relatively low in calories.

Coffee, tea, calorie-free soft drinks, bullion without fat, salt and pepper, garlic, paprika, parsley, nutmeg and cinnamon, lemon, mustard, horseradish, mint, and lime contain a negligible number of calories. Using them for salad dressings and in other creative ways is a sound and common recommendation for diabetics and people wanting to reduce calories.

Table 10   Low Fat, Low Calorie Food Alternatives

Food	Low fat alternative	Calories saved
Baked chicken with skin, ½ breast	Skin removed	40
Ground beef, 27% fat, 3 oz broiled	18% fat	90
American cheese, 1 slice	Low-fat variety	50
Sour cream, 2 tbsp	Plain yogurt	40
Cream cheese, 1 oz	Creamed cottage cheese	70
Whole milk, 1 cup	Skim	70
Potato chips, 10 large	Popcorn unbuttered 2 cups	110
Cake doughnut, 1 plain	Lightly buttered toast with ½ tsp sugar and nutmeg and cinnamon	120

Small but Frequent Feedings

A common problem for diabetics is the tendency for the blood sugar to rise too high in the first hour or two after eating. This has been the basis for limiting the number of calories consumed at each meal and spreading the calories out in the form of several snacks during the day. Whether a person has type 1 or type 2 diabetes, or is a nondiabetic, the multiple feeding schedule has several advantages as compared to eating most of your food in one, two, or three feedings per day.

The blood sugar remains more constant.   A drop in blood sugar is believed to be one factor that regulates appetite. As the time between feedings increases, blood sugar tends to drop and the appetite increases. Diabetics who have experienced insulin reaction will vouch for this. When the blood sugar level plummets as it can during an insulin reaction, the appetite becomes ravenous. A common American eating pattern is typified by a light breakfast or skipping breakfast and eating a light lunch. By midafternoon, however, as the blood sugar level decreases, the appetite rises and people are often prone to grabbing a sugar-laden snack such as a candy bar, ice cream, or soft drink, which will be rapidly digested and thus elevate the blood sugar. However, in a person whose pancreas produces insulin, quickly digested foods also quickly raise the insulin level. Normally, insulin secretion increases as the blood sugar level rises, which facilitates the passage of glucose into the tissues. Ideally, insulin secretion matches the blood sugar level so the blood sugar remains relatively constant. However, in many people a factor that determines the amount of insulin secreted is the rate at which the blood sugar level rises after eating. The faster the rise the greater the secretion of insulin. In such people, consequently, a mismatch is created in which insulin secretion exceeds the actual quantity of sugar in the blood. This results in a faster than normal removal of glucose from the blood as it passes into the tissues. Thus, the blood sugar begins to decrease and the appetite rises again. You can see how a vicious cycle can be established by not consuming adequate food at breakfast and lunch. This pattern is probably very common in many teenagers in particular. To prevent such a pattern one should eat at regular intervals throughout the day. It's no wonder that people who eat little in the first half of the day eat so much at dinner and in the evening.

Less fat is stored.   You have always believed that a calorie is a calorie. Research now indicates otherwise. For unknown reasons, consuming the same foods and same number of calories in four to six feedings per day results in less weight gain than when the food is consumed in one, two, or three feedings. This is a meaningful bit of information as it provides a pain-free, effortless way to assist in losing fat and maintaining the loss.

Serum cholesterol is reduced.   When the same amount and kinds of food are spread over four to six feedings per day rather than one or two meals, the total serum cholesterol level is less.

   In summary, large meals seem counterproductive to weight control. The eating patterns of many children again may serve as a good model. Eat moderate amounts, eat frequently and move after you have eaten.

Tasty, Low Calorie Snacks for Diabetics

Recipes abound in our diabetic magazines and newsletters. I am not going to provide an exhaustive appendix on recipes but I will share some of my longtime favorites. They are favorites because they are simple and fast to prepare, nutritious, and low in calories because they are low in sugar and fat.

Oatmeal Cookies

2 cups oatmeal (660 calories, 9-1/2 carbohydrate exchanges)
1 cup whole wheat flour (400 calories, 6 carbohydrate exchanges)
4 tbsp raisins (80 calories, 2 fruit exchanges)
1 small banana (80 calories, 2 fruit exchanges)
1 small packet of artificial sweetener (zero calories)
1/4 cup liquid vegetable oil (485 calories, 12 fat exchanges)
1 cup skim milk (90 calories, 1 milk exchange with no fat; the 2 fat exchanges in the milk exchange may be included in the vegetable oil fat exchanges)

Stir liquids; add dry contents and mix. Bake at 350° for 15 minutes.

To calculate the food exchanges for each cookie, you can add the food exchanges and divide by the number of cookies made. This allows more precision in knowing exactly what is in each cookie. For example, the total number of exchanges is:

Carbohydrate exchanges = 9-1/2 + 6 = 15-1/2
Fruit exchanges = 2 + 2 = 4
Fat exchanges = 12 minus 2 exchanges not in
    skim milk = 10
Milk exchange = 1

If you made a dozen cookies, each the same size, then the exchanges per cookie are as follows:

1-1/3 carbohydrate exchange
1/3 fruit exchange
1 fat exchange

I have rounded off my calculations to the nearest one third of an exchange. I think this allows enough accuracy. Note that I have omitted the milk exchange per cookie; this is because each cookie has less than 10% of one milk exchange. Also, the two fat exchanges not in the skim milk are accounted for by subtracting them from the fat exchanges in the vegetable oil.

While most diabetic recipe books include the food exchanges per serving, I wanted to demonstrate that it isn't too difficult to calculate food exchanges for recipes you create yourself.

Granola

Granola has the same components as the oatmeal cookies but no flour is used and the amount of water is greatly reduced. Add seeds and nuts. Bake for several hours at a very low heat; occasionally stir.

Whole Wheat Chapatis

This is an unleavened bread that is made in India and Afghanistan and takes about 6 minutes to stir up.

2 cups whole wheat flour
Enough water and liquid vegetable oil to make the mix doughy.
    (To save calories, keep the oil to a minimum.)
Handful of raisins and nuts or seeds.

Mix and bake at 350° for 15 minutes.

Blender Fruit Milkshake (Athlete's Milkshake)

One or more fruit juices
One banana, handful of strawberries
Skim milk
Ice cubes

My kids and their friends love this in the summer. I call this "The Athlete's Milkshake" because it is high in protein (from the milk) and electrolytes (minerals such as calcium, potassium and magnesium). Although it is a misconception that athletes need more protein than sedentary people, the milk gets additional calcium into your diet. Osteoporosis or bone demineralization affects a large number of women, particularly in their postmenopausal years. Many nutritionists think women should consume far more calcium than the RDA level of 800 mg. Milk is a rich source of calcium.

How Effective are Appetite Suppressants?

A summary of some 200 studies that examined the effect of appetite suppressants on weight loss indicated that the weight loss each week averaged only 1/2 pound over a period of 24 weeks. This is no more effective and perhaps is less effective than exercise alone. In addition, whereas exercise contributes to your health in a wide variety of ways, appetite suppressants usually depress central nervous function and have a tendency to make one tired, depressed, lethargic and drowsy.

Insulin and Appetite

The theory that insulin level in the blood regulates appetite is becoming increasingly substantiated by recent research evidence. Formerly it was held that the blood sugar level was the prime regulator, but current data are tending to refute this view. This may explain why diabetics who take large amounts of insulin feel hungry much of the time. It may also explain why obese people have so much difficulty cutting down on food enough to create a negative caloric intake in comparison to their energy expenditure. With more body fat, more insulin is produced because more of it is needed to promote the entry of glucose into cells. These research results clearly indicate that any factor that reduces insulin may also reduce the appetite. This obviously points to the importance of reducing body fat and increasing physical activity, because both factors reduce insulin secretion in nondiabetics and reduce the need for insulin or oral blood sugar-lowering medication in diabetics.

A second finding from the study of insulin and its effect on appetite has been that foods widely vary in the extent they raise blood insulin levels. When pure glucose is eaten, the blood sugar level rapidly rises, but then it also quickly drops as insulin is secreted. The blood insulin level, however, remains elevated for several hours. Fructose, a sugar found in fruits, causes a slower rise in blood sugar as well as insulin secretion. Table sugar or sucrose is a combination of glucose and fructose but produces a similar response as pure fructose. In one study, subjects were given a drink containing either glucose, fructose, or plain water. Two hours later all subjects were allowed to eat a buffet dinner. The fructose group consumed about 200 calories less than the water group while the glucose group ate about 250 calories more than the water group. The implication is obvious and potent: Prior to meals stay away from glucose, but purposely eat some food high in fructose. If a modification as simple as eating a piece of fruit could help you reduce 200 calories from your evening meal each day, a pound of fat could be lost every 18 days. In one year 20 pounds could be shed!

A number of foods have been tested and compared on the basis of how quickly they raise the blood sugar and blood insulin levels. Each food is thus indexed to a number with glucose having a value of 100 to serve as a baseline for comparison. Foods with a lower index cause a slower rise in blood sugar and insulin. Table 11 summarizes the glycemic index of a number of common foods.

Researchers have noted for many years that chronically obese people are more responsive to environmental cues relating to food. TV commercials and pictures in magazines elicit a stronger signal to eat in the obese than in the nonobese. Now researchers are suggesting that the reason obese people are such a soft touch is because they begin secreting extra insulin even before eating food that stimulates the appetite. One psychologist compares this conditioning to Pavlov's dog. The dog was conditioned to salivate when a bell was rung just as obese people apparently begin secreting extra insulin in response to a food cue or stimulus. The psychologist suggested that the association could be broken by purposely concentrating on a food cue such as a picture of a favorite food but not allowing oneself to eat. If repeated consistently, the experiment suggests that the insulin secretion will finally be blunted

Table 11   The Glycemic Index of Various Foods (glucose = 100)

Sugars	
Fructose	20
Sucrose	59
Honey	87
Bread, pasta, rice (spaghetti lowest, white rice highest)	47-72
Cereals (oatmeal lowest, cornflakes highest)	49-80
Fruits (apples lowest, raisins highest)	39-64
Dairy products (skim milk lowest, ice cream and yogurt highest)	32-36
Root vegetables (sweet potatoes lowest)	48-97
Peas and beans (soybeans lowest, peas highest)	15-51
Miscellaneous	
Peanuts	13
Tomato soup	38
Potato chips	51
Candy bar	68

so that the food cue will not have the effect of raising the appetite.

While all the facts are not yet in on insulin and appetite, present research does suggest that insulin may play a key role. Diabetics might well use this information to minimize the rise in blood sugar after eating. Note that oatmeal has the lowest glycemic index of the cereals tested. Because it is common for many of us who use lente and NPH insulin to have elevated blood sugar readings in the morning, I administer my morning insulin about 45 minutes before eating breakfast and I usually have oatmeal as the main source of carbohydrate for breakfast. Both factors are aimed at keeping my blood sugar normal in the morning.

Appetite and Satiety Mechanisms

We have seen from previous discussion that weight gain and weight loss are more complex than simply computing the balance between caloric intake and caloric expenditure. Multiple feedings do not add to fat stores to the same degree as when the same number of calories are consumed in one or two meals per day; foods high in fat seem to promote fat deposition as compared to a more mixed diet; some foods, depending on the speed with which they elevate blood sugar and insulin levels, increase the appetite considerably more than others. Such discoveries are helping us to understand that obese people are not simply gluttonous overeaters. A recent study adds another fact to this already complex situation: Lean people, when overfed, increase their metabolic rate, minimizing weight gain, while the metabolism of obese people remains largely unchanged. It is presently unknown if the difference is genetic in origin or if it is a developed trait. Some experts suggest that the trait of not increasing metabolism when overfed may be a genetic factor that increased the survival of people in times of famine. Thus a trait may have evolved in the species to enhance our ability to withstand limited food intake. In the United States today, possession of this trait would seemingly make obesity a certainty. The Pima Indians of Arizona may illustrate possession of this trait because as a group they have an unusually high occurrence of obesity; about 80% of all adults are obese.

Discovering the source of the metabolic problem in obese people is complex. The appetite is regulated in a portion of the brain called the appestat, a component of a structure called the hypothalamus. Activity of the appestat is triggered by several substances, each of which could be a cause of obesity if not produced or transported in proper quantity. The most widely accepted theory today holds that blood sugar level is the key to appetite control. When the blood sugar drops, the appestat signals an increase in appetite in order to cause a person to eat, which in turn will raise the blood sugar. Another chemical linked to appetite control is serotonin, a secretion of certain types of nerve cells. This nerve transmitter substance enables nerve impulses to be carried through specific nerve pathways in the brain. When the brain is relatively low in serotonin, the appetite is increased. Carbohydrates tend to keep serotonin levels in the brain relatively high and therefore the appetite is depressed. So, serotonin and blood sugar appear to be related in affecting appetite.

Exercise generally reduces appetite because of its effect on the blood sugar and serotonin levels. Exercise stimulates the secretion of the "fight or flight" hormones by the adrenal gland. These hormones cause the liver to release glucose in an attempt to keep the blood sugar level adequate for normal brain function and to supply extra fuel if needed to the active muscles. By maintaining the blood sugar level, the appestat and all other portions of the brain receive adequate fuel. Exercise also increases serotonin production.

In addition, the adrenal "fight or flight" hormones released during exercise mobilize fat or take some fat from storage and move it into the blood. The longer a person exercises, the greater the rise in blood fats, which also means that active muscles begin to preferentially use more and more fat in releasing energy. That is why carbohydrate in muscle tissue becomes less and less used as an energy source as the duration of activity increases. Consequently, to move stored fat into the bloodstream and to allow fat to become the prevalent source of energy in a workout, long sessions at moderate to low intensity are best. Long-distance athletes become very efficient in their ability to carry out these fat metabolism processes. One notable result of endurance training is a body that likes to burn fat and consequently, one that does not store much of it. Caffeine is also known to enhance the utilization of fat as an energy source during exercise. One recently published study showed that fat loss was significantly enhanced in a group of rats that were given caffeine prior to their daily exercise. The fat loss was significant in the rats that exercised but were not given caffeine, but the combination of the two produced greater overall fat loss. We know that caffeine promotes fat usage in animals and some studies show the same results in humans.

Exercise, therefore, has a potent effect on appetite that can last for several hours. It is not presently known if these training effects described, as well as the acute effect of a single exercise session on the appetite, work in the obese as well as the normal individual. It would appear, however, that sedentary obese people may be particularly ripe for making major metabolic changes. With exercise of relatively moderate intensity but prolonged duration, the obese may be capable of a metabolic transformation aimed at becoming more similar to endurance athletes. Training studies in nonobese normal subjects indicate that these metabolic changes occur in several weeks of appropriate training.

So far, we have discussed current theories of appetite control. The other side of the coin deals with satiety or reaching a satisfied state that makes us stop eating. Current theory suggests that the insulin level in the cerebrospinal fluid around the brain and spinal cord determines satiety (whereas insulin level in the blood seems to be a factor controlling appetite). That is, once the insulin level in this fluid rises to a set level, we no longer wish to continue eating. However, insulin levels in the blood and cerebrospinal fluid do not rise as soon as we begin eating. First, the food must be digested and the glucose formed from the breakdown of carbohydrate digestion passes into the bloodstream. Then, additional insulin is secreted into the blood and, in theory, the insulin level in the cerebrospinal fluid rises. These events typically require about 5 to 20 minutes, depending on the mixture of foods eaten. This means that you will not necessarily feel satisfied after eating a quick meal lasting 10 or 15 minutes unless you consume a considerable volume of food. Therefore, one should eat slowly or do something immediately after having eaten that gets you away from the kitchen and eating area. Vacuum a carpet, walk the dog, or play with the kids. It is no wonder that people often nibble after a meal as they clean the kitchen and put away leftovers. You would do better to avoid the temptation and do other chores first and then return 10 to 15 minutes later and clean the table and kitchen. At that time, you should no longer feel hungry.

A second theory of satiety holds that a chemical called cholecystokinin strongly affects the sensation of satiety. This substance is secreted by the small intestine when fat enters it. The blood carries the hormone to the gall bladder, causing the gall bladder to contract rhythmically and squirt bile into the small intestine. Bile then helps to simplify fats so they can be digested and absorbed into the blood. Researchers found that a genetically obese breed of rats had below normal levels of cholecystokinin in their brains. When they injected the chemical into the rats and in later experiments, humans, the rats immediately stopped eating and the human subjects reported feeling full. While I cannot suggest any immediate application of this finding, it is interesting and again makes one appreciate the complexity of obesity.

One encouraging report came from a study in which bulky, filling foods were compared to rich, high caloric, non-filling foods as to the caloric consumption and satiety. The first diet was high in complex carbohydrates such as fruits, vegetables, and breads and low in fat. The second diet consisted of high fat meats, creamed potatoes, cake, and similar foods. When eating the bulky complex carbohydrates the caloric intake averaged 1,570 calories, but on the rich, fatty diet about 3,000 calories were consumed. The subjects, however, reported feeling equally full on both diets 3 hours after eating and the following morning. Eating the complex foods also required about 33% more time than eating the rich refined meals, which the investigators believed may be a factor in satiety. As mentioned previously, perhaps the longer meal time allowed the insulin level in the cerebrospinal fluid to rise and signal satiety. Anyway, these results are encouraging and certainly offer some potential for weight control.

After analyzing factors that possibly control appetite and satiety, it appears that exercise is beneficial because it expends calories, can improve the ability of the body to mobilize and burn fat during activity, and can reduce the appetite. A certain minimum level of physical activity seems to allow the appestat to carry out its designed function whereas a highly sedentary lifestyle is either going to make a person overweight or force many people to be hungry and perhaps nutritionally deficient for the rest of their lives.

Summary

It appears likely that the human species evolved as an organism that depended on considerable bodily movement for survival and development. For some 3 to 4 million years the pattern of activity may have become imprinted in our genes as did the evolvement of a gastrointestinal-chemical system geared at digesting grains, fruits, vegetables, meat, fish, and a variety of other foods. Only very recently in our evolution has an abrupt change in these habits occurred. People have been given the possibility of minimizing movement and significant use of the skeletal muscles and heart muscle. Foods are available in untold quantity and in concentrated caloric form. What are the results of these changes? Will the wisdom and knowledge developing today and in the future suggest a partial return to simpler ways? For the vast majority of overweight people, it does seem that relatively moderate changes in exercise and diet may normalize body fatness. As a result, people with diabetes are typically able to dramatically reduce the amount of insulin and blood sugar-lowering medication taken.

part III

Putting it All Together

chapter 10

Adapting to Stress

The purpose of this chapter is to make the reader aware that the level of happiness, enjoyment, and productivity in life is to a large degree affected by the way we react to stress. In diabetics, stress can lead to a rise or fall in blood sugar, which in turn interferes with the capacity to function optimally. It is presently unknown why stress can either raise or lower the blood sugar in diabetics. Consequently, it is difficult to anticipate how we should alter our diabetic management. Most of us probably learn that the best basis for coping with possible changes in blood sugar is to assess the blood sugar more frequently at such times. If this is not done, a vicious cycle can be established that is difficult to escape. Because we cannot typically run away from stress, the ability to learn stress-coping skills becomes of major importance in our quality of life. A key concept in this chapter is that people can learn to adapt to stressors in their lives and still be productive. Stress adaptation techniques do not require giving up an active, busy, challenging career. To some people, the mere thought of such would be stressful. Coping techniques such as meditation or yoga are sometimes mistakenly thought to be entities unto themselves. Actually, specific coping techniques should be viewed as components in a larger plan of life, one that includes an overall healthy lifestyle. The techniques can be of no value whatsoever unless they are practiced. Coping skills can dwindle away if not used, but they can be potent tools if they are practiced regularly and used at appropriate times.

What Is Stress?

Stress is the psychological stimulation associated with an event. The event may be real or imagined, and physical or psychological. Worrying about a coming exam or fretting about a meeting in which you will make a presentation are very real stressors that evoke the same biological changes (e.g., rapidly beating heart, sweating, rise in blood pressure) as those produced if you were confronted on a street by a robber. The same events, however, also occur when we experience great enjoyment and happiness. Even exercise invokes these events. Obviously these latter types of stress are positive because they make us feel better. Therefore, not all stress is bad. If you are able to adjust to the stressor and improve yourself in some way, then stress has had a beneficial effect. Probably most students experience stress when taking an exam, but if they master the test and achieve a pleasing grade, they have been successful and they feel good about themselves. Stress leading to positive changes is called eustress or positive stress.

Stress is largely based on an individual's attitudes and perceptions regarding specific events. Secretary A might be stressed to learn that she will undergo several days of training to learn how to use a computer, whereas secretary B is excited about the opportunity to learn a new skill. One person views the change as a threat, whereas the other views it in a positive way, as a challenge. Therein lies the difference. Furthermore, each secretary's capacity to learn to use the computer will probably be strongly affected by these attitudes. Stress, then, affects not only the process, that is, how we feel while performing, but also the product or the extent to which we effectively perform. It used to be believed that being an executive meant contending with high stress and poor health, but research evidence shows quite the opposite. A study of business executives listed in *Who's Who in America* in the early 1950s indicated that this group had a 30% lower death rate than a control group of nonexecutives. In another study of more than 1000 executives from companies listed in Fortune's 500, the mortality rate was only 58% as high as executives whose companies were not listed. These results clearly demonstrate that many of the executives "at the top" are able to cope with the stress of their jobs. The coping ability or adaptability may largely depend on their perception of the work as it did with the secretaries.

Several studies have related personality type to heart disease. The now well-known personality categories of type A and type B are used to describe the ambitious, impatient striver constantly on the rush, type A, and the more relaxed, take everything easy type person, type B. The classification is probably an oversimplification. One authority adds credence to this possibility by stating that our first 11 presidents lived to an average age of 81 and none of them had a heart attack. From Woodrow Wilson through Lyndon Johnson, six of the nine presidents had cardiovascular disease. It is hard to believe that our first eleven presidents were type Bs while many of those in the 20th century have been type A. The point is, the nature of the job seems to be less predictive of stress than the person's ability to cope with the job. The earlier presidents may have had healthier lifestyles such as more physical activity, absence of cigarette smoking, and a diet lower in fat. The Japanese as a society are probably even more type A than American society, yet the former have remarkably low incidence of cardiovascular disease. Again, attitudes and lifestyle may possibly explain the difference.

We tend to think of stress and its biological-psychological effects as having only negative consequences, but actually the stress mechanism has served as a key survival mechanism in human evolution. The net effect of the biological changes induced by stress provides a greater ability to do extreme physical work. Some use the term "fight or flight" response to describe this state. Our strength and endurance are increased, the blood clots very rapidly minimizing blood loss if injured, and breathing and sweating are rapidly increased. These changes allowed people to fight for hours in hand to hand combat with a sword and spear when under normal conditions they would be exhausted in several minutes by such work.

People survived extremes in the elements and deprivation of food and water because of the stress mechanism. We hear of ordinary people performing such unusual feats as lifting a car or tractor off a person. The stress mechanism was probably so critical to survival of the species that it became strongly entrenched in our genes. It was a trait that was probably strengthened through survival of those who had the greatest capacity to withstand such physical stressors.

Today most of us in Western society do not face the extreme physical dangers our ancestors did but we do still possess the stress mechanism because it is locked into our genetic code. Consequently, we react to any stressor exactly as if it required a tremendous surge of energy. We show the same rise in blood sugar and blood fat, heart rate, blood pressure, sweating, and so on. Until the 20th century these changes were usually helpful in responding to an emergency, but today they are not always helpful to us as we sit stewing in our own juices worrying about the future. If stress is chronic, the chemical changes elicited can produce high blood pressure, ulcers, cardiovascular disease and many other damaging chronic medical states. Our primitive ancestors probably didn't sit, brood and become overanxious and sick because of the stress in life. They moved, fought, and exerted strenuously in their struggle to survive. As a result of these physical efforts, the stress hormones adrenaline and noradrenaline released by the adrenal glands return to normal and the triggering effect of the hormones is stopped.

Acute stress can therefore be used to help us achieve. It may provide the energy to study many hours for an exam or prepare for a speech; it helps the athlete and entertainer to be emotionally aroused to a level where quality performance is more likely to occur and in special events, to peak or maximize performance. If we lost the ability to perceive some events in our lives as stressful, we would likely be more consistent in performance yet far less likely and far less frequently able to achieve truly outstanding performance. It would seem that the ability to perceive stress is a very basic human trait. I hate to think of what life would be like if we didn't possess the trait.

So there is a good side to stress. Every challenge and change in life creates some stress. When we jump for joy, hug someone, see a "moving" drama on television or at the movies, get a promotion, or win a ball game we experience stress as a positive event. The same biological changes occur as when we might be fighting for our lives. To be human is to have feelings that allow us to perceive various emotional states from grief to exhilaration. So, while it may seem beneficial to remove the stress in our lives, it would probably make life so boring we would have nothing to look forward to and we would never experience the highs that make life so attractive. So, with the good comes the bad; with happiness comes sadness. The trick is to achieve a balance between positive stress and negative stress. Realize, too, that it is entirely normal to experience highs and lows, and confidence as well as insecurity.

While these statements hold true for anyone, they are particularly noteworthy for a person with diabetes because effective diabetic control is determined by blood sugar and stress can affect blood sugar, which in turn can hinder our emotional state. Optimal diabetic management should include a knowledge of this bond between emotions and blood sugar and should include training in the ways to cope with emotional states triggered by stress.

The American Work Ethic and Stress

Our society was founded in part by a philosophy of hard work. The Puritan work ethic remains ingrained in our lifestyle today. We quantify many aspects of our work and even our play. "More is better" is a guide to our economy, national budget, and gross national product. Business, government, and political leaders seem to understand quite well that most people can produce more if they simply work more hours and concentrate more fully while they work. It is common and even expected in some social circles to brag about how many hours people work, how many service activities they work with, and all the things they do for their children. As with most things, a point probably exists for each of us where "more" becomes too much and we reduce the quality of our overall efforts. To be recognized in your field of work by your peers is admirable and is perhaps needed to some degree, but it is a common problem in our society to let our ambitions become excessive. The result often leads to frustration, anxiety, and reduced health.

This problem is compounded by the multiple roles most people assume. Roles may include parent, spouse, worker, or member of church, school, and community groups. If you set an unrealistic goal to be an exemplary model in each role you play it may make you less happy overall and less productive in some key aspects of your life. It may trigger a reaction that puts you into psychic overdrive, the old "work even harder" routine. If you find yourself talking faster, moving faster, forgetting things, and always concerned or preoccupied with tomorrow, then you are demonstrating excessive behavior and are probably receiving much of your extra energy via the stress mechanism. Several thousand years ago there must have been such types of people because Socrates stated his now famous quote, "Moderation in all things." This could well be a principle for healthful living as it seemingly applies to eating, exercise, work, sleep, and drinking, as well as stress.

Researchers in a number of fields have found that this principle of moderation holds true for many facets of life. They use the term the "inverted U" phenomenon, shown in Figure 10. For example, in order to obtain a conditioning effect of the cardiovascular system, we have to exert ourselves to at least 50% of our maximum oxygen uptake level. People can exert within a broad level up to maximum in order to derive an increasingly greater conditioning response. However, if most people were to consistently exert near their maximum, they would tend to suffer muscle pulls, reduced motivation to train, and finally they would quit exercising so intensely. So, the optimum training is not to go all-out each training session. Most of the training even for Olympic athletes is comprised of moderate work. What about vitamins? We know that more

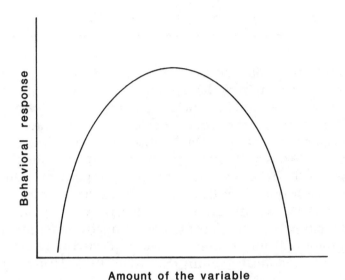

Figure 10   The inverted U phenomenon

than 40 nutrients are essential to prevent various disease states. The RDA for vitamin C is 60 mg; this provides a level well beyond that needed to prevent scurvy. Does it hold that 10 or 20 times that much will provide extra benefits such as prevention of colds? Researchers say no. Interestingly, it seems that when people take megadosages of vitamins and minerals (10 times or more the recommended amount), absorption of other nutrients is impaired. Although one may be expecting and hoping for added health, quite the opposite may actually occur.

Does it seem logical then that extra work most days of your life will likely make you more productive or happier or healthier? Is it best for you as well as those significant others to attempt to be a role model needed for others in all facets of your life? The principle of moderation is so simple that it is commonly overlooked. I doubt we need the confirmation provided by research to convince most of us that too much of anything winds up being destructive in the long run.

How Do I Start?

To live a balanced life and one that allows you to be productive yet happy with your home life and yourself requires setting priorities and then holding to moderation. Take paper and pencil and write down the key concerns you have within each major role you play in life. List being diabetic as a role because of its impact on all other facets of your life and because it is a part of you that requires planning and thought each day of your life. Within each role, rank the order of your concerns. Next rank each role. This is an interesting and challenging task, and I recommend doing it whenever you feel symptoms of being chronically overburdened or overstressed or your behavior is becoming excessive. Table 12 gives an example of one woman's major roles and concerns about each.

Going through the task in written fashion and rank ordering forces you to sort out where you wish to head in life. It tends to prompt action. The actual doing of it may itself be initially stressful but often a sense of inner peace results. We all have wishes and frustrations, and the first step to achieve, or reduce them as the case may be, is to identify them. Obviously the next step is to do something. I would suggest tackling no more than two or three concerns at a time, but first prioritize among them, or at least select the two or three that presently bother you the most. Then you will tend to feel better as you take a positive step toward progress; that alone should boost your spirits. Achievement regarding these concerns is now your challenge.

Learning to Say "No"

I am basically a "yes" man and have always found it difficult to say no to someone. I think it may be a fear of what others may think about me—"he's selfish," "he's lazy," or "he doesn't care about the organization." For most of us, I

Table 12   Major Concerns of a Hypothetical Woman

Role	Rank order	Major concerns
Mother	1	Want to spend more time with children in peaceful, relaxing situations
	3	Want children to do household chores without griping and without having to be reminded repeatedly
	2	Would like to see children read more and watch TV less
Spouse	1	Spend more meaningful time alone with husband: talk more frequently, quiet dinner.
	2	Have husband more actively help discipline children
Diabetic	1	Achieve a tighter control of blood sugar
	2	Call insurance company about coverage of glucometer
	3	Need to get active, fit, and lose weight
Self	1	Lose weight
	2	Want to finish my bachelor's degree
	3	Would love to get out and play tennis again this spring and summer on a regular basis
President, PTA	1	Want to get more parents involved and make a real contribution to the school
	2	Husband needs to help me here
Den Mother, Cub Scouts	1	Plan for next month's honors award dinner
	2	Need to get Mrs. Smith on the ball: She's not doing her share

suspect, learning to say no is not an easy thing. However, I have improved a lot. I have found that when I mention I am unable to do something because I am committed to spending time with my family, not many will argue the point. They may even respect the comment. Family is still a highly respected word in our society. However, even the comment, "I'd like to but I just can't at this time" is a nice general statement, which diplomatically gets you off the hook. You, too, can learn to say no and I think it helps immensely to have a plan for doing so.

A second point about saying no is that we have to admit that if we say no, it is not the end of the world for the other party. No matter who you are or what your qualifications, there are other people who can provide the service being asked of you. Pass the buck: Mention a colleague or friend who can provide the same service. It is not a dirty trick as they can say no, too. I am asked to speak to business and civic groups frequently about fitness, diabetes, weight loss, and stress management, and I have given more than 350 such presentations in my career. However, because I like and expect to make presentations at my own professional meetings, I have to limit my presentations to nonprofessional groups. When someone calls my office and requests that I speak, I indicate a need to check my calendar. I see what other events are happening in my life that week and that month and make a decision. This pause usually gives me enough time to assess the real importance of this request. After this brief reflection, I find it easier to reject the offer if I wish. I may say something like "Oh, I'd really enjoy doing that but my calendar says I'm booked up." I may follow with the name of a colleague who could speak. Anyway, I have yet to have anyone question my calendar. Furthermore, I have certain policies I follow; for instance, I simply will not speak during final exam week. My ego enjoys hearing how much a particular group would like to hear me speak, but their enjoyment is secondary to my health, happiness and feeling of control.

Symptoms of Stress

Symptoms of stress appear in everyone occasionally but when the following symptoms linger and become chronic, appropriate remedial steps should be taken.

1. Continual mental and physical fatigue that doesn't respond to rest
2. Depression
3. Irritability
4. Decreased self-esteem and self-confidence
5. Decreased interest in sex
6. Difficulty in concentration
7. Insomnia, especially early in the morning

Recognition of these symptoms is not difficult but doing something about them is the critical ameliorative step.

Coping Techniques

A number of techniques can be used to reduce acute stress. I feel, however, that stress coping procedures are most effective if one employs a daily pattern that includes quiet, relaxing, peaceful activities. These may include light exercise such as walking or yoga, reading, sitting and thinking, crocheting, or praying. These activities should be done purely for their enjoyment and sense of relaxation, and they should not be activities thought of as productive or efficient. I think of such activities as being part of the foundation for mental health and hence part of a person's foundation for coping with stress. These activities should be done daily to act as a cushion to the stress of everyday living. If performed daily minor stressors will not tend to become major stressors, stress can be dissipated, and when major stressors do appear, your adaptational energy will be higher and you will be better able to cope with the problem. So, as with most health habits, your daily activities are the most important determinants of your stress coping ability. While learning special stress management techniques such as visualization or meditation helps to adjust to an acute stressor, I feel that your daily habits as regards stress control are more important than special techniques used only in times of stress. Also, unless you practice these activities or skills frequently, you will probably not be able to use them effectively when stress levels are high. Research indicates that anxiety and stress are reduced only for several hours after various coping techniques are used. This further illustrates the need for the practice of stress-reducing strategies on a daily or even several times per day basis.

The body responds similarly to each of the coping strategies to be described. The effects include decreased muscle tension; reduced blood pressure, heart rate, and metabolic rate; a change in brain wave activity to a lesser state of arousal; and a psychological sense of being more relaxed and peaceful. The techniques can help one relax before a stressing event such as taking an exam, playing a big ballgame, and making a speech. They can also be used to unwind after a stressing event. The key is that in order for most of them to be effective, they must be practiced. Unless you develop a skill in using the techniques and psychologically are willing or receptive, they will be limited in helping you.

Physical Activity

Exercise is nature's antistress mechanism. People have realized for many years that physical exertion has a beneficial effect on the mind. The ancient Athenian ideal of "mens sana in corpore sano" or "a healthy mind in a healthy body" expresses this relationship. Similarly, most of us have experienced the positive effect on our emotions after a stressful incident by taking a walk and "working off some steam." Researchers have provided experimental evidence that exercise helps us psychologically and today is used in treating a number of psychiatric disorders. Exercise has been used in psychiatric medicine as a therapeutic tool since before World War II at the world famous Menninger Clinic in Topeka, Kansas. At recent meetings of the American Psychological Association, experts have presented evidence as to the psychologic values of exercise. One authority, Thaddeus Kostrubala, has even written a book for his colleagues explaining how his use of jogging was used to counsel patients. His approach is noteworthy because he jogs with his patients and counsels them on the run instead of on the couch.

The biochemical basis for the effects of exercise on the psyche is being unraveled and better understood. Central nervous system secretions such as beta endorphins and norepinephrine are believed by some researchers to provide the sense of relaxation and elevation in mood following exercise. Even the "runners' high," the heightened sensation of tranquility and energy experienced by runners at times, has been theorized to be caused by the beta endorphins. Exercise can also provide an opportunity to be alone, which in itself may be relaxing. Many stimuli in the work environment such as telephone calls, people, memos, meetings and deadlines exaggerate the state of arousal as well as the duration we are aroused. As we move, talk and try to think more rapidly in response to these multiple stimuli, the tissues in general are overstimulated by the sympathetic nervous system. We may or may not notice the tension creeping into the shoulders, lower back, and back of neck. The stress mechanism is in operation and it is trying to help us accomplish our many tasks. If we remove ourselves from the environment and focus or concentrate on a single thought, we can reduce this state of neural and hormonal overdrive and thus the attendant symptoms. Consequently, exercise may allow us or force us to concentrate on other things. While playing racquetball or any game, concentration is obviously placed on aspects of the game itself rather than aspects of your job. While exercising outdoors the beauty of the environment may call a person's attention. Many joggers feel that the repetitive sound of each step and their own rhythmic breathing tend to place them in a trance-like state. Whatever actually happens, the mind is left relatively undisturbed and free, which may provide a basis for feeling relaxed and renewed. No wonder many runners feel they do some of their best thinking while running. Many great writers and philosophers were known to be great walkers. Perhaps these simple, repetitive activities allow the brain a relatively lengthy time to exist in a free or unencumbered state.

An improved state of physical fitness usually involves weight loss, a more pleasing physical appearance, and more energy. Such changes likely provide a sense of accomplishment, sometimes even a sense of being more youthful or physically superior to others of the same age. All such states are bound to make a person feel better about oneself and to promote a sense of confidence. Years of research have also indicated that in animals and man, physically trained organisms can tolerate more stress of nearly any type. In other words, fit people have a higher breaking point. The purpose of stress management and living a balanced life, however, is not to see how much stress you can tolerate before you keel over or become ill, but it is to prevent stress from ever reaching a high level, which if sustained long enough will cause illness or disease. One study compared the effects of walking and jogging to the three leading prescription medications used in treating anxiety. The exercise was just as effective as the drugs and of course it provided a higher level of fitness than taking the medication. A study performed in our laboratory compared the amount of several stress hormones secreted during exercise in people having different fitness levels. The elevation of adrenaline and other hormones in the more fit subjects was markedly lower than in the less fit subjects. Also, the least fit subject had the highest rise in adrenaline secretion, whereas the most fit subject had the lowest rise. Other researchers have found that aerobic training reduces the level of adrenaline stored in the heart. Those with large stores of adrenaline in the heart muscle are more prone to abnormal heart rhythm, so training provides a safety mechanism that reduces the tendency for this condition. So, even highly fit people should be concerned with stress. Exercise itself is a stress; if applied for a reasonable time and intensity with adequate time for recovery, the organism is strengthened and somewhat inured to stress. However, exercise beyond a point can be destructive. Injuries can result and even immune function suffers, leaving an overly tired athlete ripe for illness. As previously stated, moderation is the key.

The key to using exercise as a stress coping technique is to select one or more activities that can be used consistently every week and every month for the rest of your life. The activities should include some that develop and maintain aerobic fitness. I like to encourage a variety of physical activity because of weather, facility and equipment limitations, and because if one is injured, it is nice to have an alternative form of fitness exercise. Runners can particularly understand this. Many die-hard runners become very dissatisfied, frustrated and even stressed when unable to run. I have known many injured joggers who were mildly depressed while waiting for an injury to heal. Runners would probably be wise to alternate running at least twice a week with some other more gentle form of exercise such as walking, cross-country skiing, cycling, or swimming. Runners would probably experience far fewer injuries and not become so dependent on running.

Realize that exercise can be psychologically stressing if we become overly competitive with ourselves or other people. Golfers and tennis players have been known to break clubs and racquets; some runners become obsessed with trying to run a distance in a certain time or to run so many miles each week. All of these are examples of excessive behavior that probably elevate stress rather than minimize it.

Glasser wrote a book titled *Positive Addiction*. In it he described how people can become addicted to positive aspects of life. To become addicted to exercise he stated that the activity should possess the following characteristics:

1. Be noncompetitive
2. Require minimal skill
3. Provide positive feedback within several sessions
4. Not require other people
5. Have inherent value
6. Allow rapid progress in terms of performing the activity
7. Minimize the likelihood of self-criticism

I believe Glasser's criteria are valid as well as realistic. I have often thought about reasons that explain why some people such as myself exercise all of their lives and why when people begin a fitness program, some drop out whereas others develop and maintain the habit. These criteria, from my viewpoint, are excellent and I urge you to relate them carefully to activities you think you may wish to do.

Deep Breathing

Go to a quiet spot, sit comfortably, and concentrate on your breathing. It sounds simple and it is. Close your eyes and feel the air move into your nostrils as you inspire. To enhance concentration, imagine that as the air enters your body it is a soft yellowish color that illuminates the airways as you breathe. Try to breathe slowly and deeply; let your tummy expand slightly outward as you inspire and mentally watch the yellow haze enter your chest and sink low into the abdomen. Feel the warmth of the golden air as it pleasantly, naturally, effortlessly fills your lungs. Visualize and feel the air leave the lungs, airways, and finally the nostrils. Repeat the cycle mentally a dozen or more times.

Even if on your initial attempts you can maintain attention only a dozen times or so, you will probably feel a sense of calmness pervade you. After a moment's pause, repeat another cycle of a dozen or so slow, deep, and relaxed breaths emphasizing seeing and feeling the golden, warm air. The procedure of alternating phases of concentration with pauses is similar to doing weight training. After performing a number of movements, you pause to rest and then execute more movements. If you do this deep breathing routine once or twice a day you will most likely find that you will soon be able to focus on more breaths before you feel the need to pause, and by maintaining yourself in this relaxed state for a longer period while deep breathing, you should get more out of each session.

Progressive Muscle Relaxation

This technique was developed in the 1930s by a physician named Edmund Jacobson. It involves alternately tensing and relaxing local muscle groups. As with any relaxation strategy, it is simple (it has to be or you wouldn't be able to relax while doing it) and it is best performed in a quiet atmosphere with the eyes closed. The ideal posture to assume is lying on your back with a pillow or two under the knees to keep the knees bent, which prevents arching and tightening the lower back. Place a pillow under your head as well. Remember that the idea is not to fall asleep but to stay awake and focus attention on various muscle groups. The procedure can certainly be done while sitting comfortably although lying probably encourages a greater state of relaxation.

Start by pushing just the toes against the sole of your shoes. Start with a small amount of force and over 5 or 6 seconds gradually increase the force to near maximum. Then slowly decrease the tension back to a baseline of zero tension or complete relaxation. I like to visualize in my mind a line on a graph rising gradually to a peak and then slowly ebbing to the base or horizontal axis. Figure 11 depicts this visualization. After the contraction, imagine the toes to be limp, heavy and utterly relaxed. They should feel so heavy that they want to droop downward. Go back and visualize the baseline on the graph; imagine it to be a straight line nearly touching the horizontal axis. Keep it there for several seconds. Now begin to push the toes into the soles a second time and gradually build to a peak. Hold the peak level a second or two and then allow the tension to diminish slowly to zero.

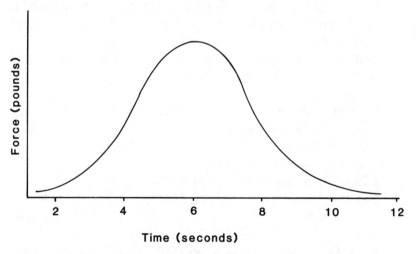

Figure 11 Visualization of the increasing and decreasing force during progressive muscle relaxation

This cycle of contraction and relaxation for a given group of muscles can be performed several times. I think two cycles per muscle is enough to train your mind to control local muscle tension and it is brief enough to allow you to work most of the large muscles of the body. I favor beginning with the toes and then working upward as follows:

1. Toes
2. Calves (back of the lower leg)
3. Quadriceps (frontal thigh muscles)
4. Glutei (buttocks)
    The contractile action here is one of pinching the buttocks together as if squeezing and holding a penny in place.
5. Lower back
    Tense the lower back muscles isometrically (that is, without actually moving the spine). Think of trying to bend backward but resist the movement by tensing the abdominal muscles.
6. Upper back
    The movement in this area is a squeezing of the shoulder blades together.
7. Trapezius (the muscle sloping downward and outward to the top of the shoulder from the upper back of the neck and skull)
    This movement consists of raising or shrugging the shoulders upward toward the ears.
8. Front of arms
    Contract the biceps isometrically without actually moving the arms as if you were a body-builder showing off your biceps.
9. Fingers, chest and upper body
    Place the fingertips of each hand together so that they slightly touch. Squeeze the fingers together but do not allow the arms or shoulders to move. Many muscles, both large and small, are activated in this exercise including those of the fingers, forearms, arms, shoulders, chest, and latissimus dorsi (the large muscles below the arm pit that sweep across the back and side of the rib cage).

10. Forehead
Here all you have to do is wrinkle the brow.

Obviously, other muscle groups and even individual muscles could be added to this sequence. The 10 listed, however, include most of the major muscles of the body.

Visualization

Simply said, visualization is dreaming while you are awake. The idea is to create an image in your mind of a peaceful, serene environment such as gently swinging in a hammock on a beautiful day. Focus on details to make it seem as real and vivid as possible. For example, imagine that you have cut the lawn, that you did several other chores earlier in the day, and you now have several hours ahead completely free to relax. You will be alone for several hours and you are now going to lean back in the hammock with a cold glass of lemonade, and just relax. The smooth, rhythmic swaying is so relaxing. Your muscles are relaxed and you feel pleasantly tired from your lawn mowing. The sky overhead is a cloudless, beautiful, deep blue; the green leaves overhead, the thick trimmed hedges, and shrubbery make this spot in your backyard a perfect place to relax. You breathe a deep sigh and feel yourself sink into the hammock. It feels so good. Life is so good. The world seems so tranquil. It feels good to be alive and it feels good to be surrounded by nature in this peaceful and verdant spot.

Practicing this technique will enhance your ability to embellish the image you create. The key, I believe, is to make the scene so real that your nervous system believes you are actually there. If this works, the activity of the nervous system is diminished. You are taken out of an arousal state and you are gradually moved to a state of tranquility. As a result, your heart rate and breathing rate slow, muscle tension decreases, and so on. Other images amenable to creating this state are sitting on a mountain top, sitting beside a mountain lake, and lying in warm sand on a beach.

Yoga Stretching

It is beyond the purpose here to discuss yoga in its broad sense of being a philosophy of life. For our purposes, discussion is limited to it as a form of relaxation.

The important trait of yoga that makes it effective as a means of relaxation is that it is performed very slowly. When this characteristic is applied to a variety of movements it makes yoga or any slow stretch effective in developing flexibility as well as enhancing relaxation. Several movements are described below. They have been selected because they promote relaxation in general but also because they reduce local muscle tension in areas where muscles commonly tighten. Many other specific exercises and postures are used by advocates of this type of exercise.

The essential instruction in each exercise below is to perform the movements with extreme slowness.

Neck roll.   Begin by lowering the chin to the chest. Slowly turn the head toward one shoulder; make the motion so slow as to make it appear you are moving in superslow motion. When you reach the shoulder and begin the movement backwards, do not push or exert much force backward as this may tighten the muscles crossing the back of the neck. Instead, let the flexibility of your neck and state of muscle tension determine how far backward the head moves but do not attempt to make this an exercise in flexibility. You should feel as though your neck is rolling smoothly at a constant speed in a circular orbit. Take at least 15 seconds to complete one revolution. Do several circles and then switch directions.

After completing this exercise, sit or stand erect and focus on the degree of relaxation achieved. You should feel considerably looser in the neck and shoulders, which should enhance your overall sense of relaxation. This is a great exercise to use when you have been immobile for several hours such as driving, typing, writing, or reading. It really gets the kinks out of the neck.

Forward bend. Ordinarily I don't recommend standing toe touch-like movements because they tend to be hard on the back, but this one does not require going all the way down and some modifications are made so that most people can perform this exercise without discomfort. Bend the knees slightly and let both arms hang limp in front of you. Very slowly, bend forward while keeping the arms in the same position, and maintain the knees in a bent position throughout. Also, tighten the tummy muscles throughout the exercise to reduce the strain on the lower back. Continue bending until the hands are just below the knees. Now gently move the torso from side to side several times. If you are quite relaxed, the arms will sway from side to side even after the torso has stopped moving. At about the same speed you lowered the trunk, raise yourself to the starting position.

This exercise relaxes the entire length of the back as well as the arms and shoulders. It is effective in times of stress but also for relaxing tight, overused muscles after strenuous work or exercise. After I shovel snow or rake leaves, this exercise is very effective in relaxing tight, stiff muscles.

Many other movements can be used depending on what muscular regions you wish to relax. I like these two because they treat muscles many of us commonly find tight and they relax so much of our total musculature.

Effect of Diet and Drugs on Stress

A number of foods and drugs used by millions of Americans on a daily basis stimulate the secretion of the stress hormones. Obviously, if you are trying to reduce stress and the sense of rush and hurry in your life, these chemicals should be used judiciously.

Any factor causing a rapid drop in blood sugar will stimulate stress hormone secretion by the adrenal gland. Consequently, the glycemic index becomes a factor related to stress as does the close observation of a diabetic's blood sugar level. Foods with a high glycemic index rapidly elevate the blood sugar, which tends to promote an excess secretion of insulin in nondiabetics. The excess insulin leads to a rapid drop in blood sugar, triggering the adrenal glands to secrete adrenalin. The result is a hungry person in a food-induced state of stress. Figure 12 portrays these events. To minimize this possible source of stress nondiabetics could eat foods such as candy, sugar and sugared beverages after a meal rather than on an empty stomach. In eating a typical meal, these effects are greatly reduced by the contribution of other foods with a lower glycemic index. For those of us with diabetes, simply letting our blood sugar drop too low or too high can cause the secretion of the adrenal stress hormones making us feel anxious and irritable. All other things being equal, when the blood sugar is reasonably close to normal, we tend to feel best emotionally and psychologically.

Caffeine and nicotine also stimulate the adrenal glands. The most common sources of caffeine are coffee, soft drinks, tea, chocolate, and over-the-counter drugs such as appetite suppressants, cold remedies, diuretics, and pain relievers. Table 13 summarizes the amount of caffeine in these sources.

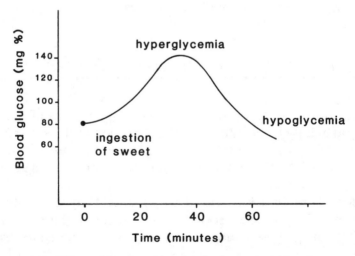

Figure 12   Effect of foods with a high glycemic index (e.g., sugar, candy) on the blood sugar level of nondiabetics

Table 13   Common Sources of Caffeine[1]

Source	Caffeine (mg)
Coffee	
Drip (5 oz)	146
Percolated (5 oz)	110
Instant, regular (5 oz)	53
Decaffeinated (5 oz)	2
Tea	
1-minute brew (5 oz)	9 to 33
3-minute brew (5 oz)	20 to 46
5-minute brew (5 oz)	20 to 50
Canned ice tea (12 oz)	22 to 36
Soft drinks	
Regular colas	
Pepsi-Cola	43
Royal Crown	40
Cocoa-Cola	40
Diet colas	
Diet Rite	42
Diet Coke	48
Diet Pepsi	38
Tab	48
Pepsi Light	38
Caffeine-free regular colas	
Coke	0
Shasta Free	0
Pepsi Free	0
Like	0
RC 100	0
Caffeine-free diet colas	
RC 100	0
Pepsi Free	0
Diet Coke	0
Like	0
Shasta Free	0
Tab	0
Cocoa and chocolate	
Cocoa beverage (water mix, 6 oz)	10
Milk chocolate (1 oz)	6
Baking chocolate (1 oz)	35

(Cont.)

Table 13   (Cont.)

Source	Caffeine (mg)
Nonprescription drugs	
Stimulants (standard dose)	
Caffedrine capsules	200
NoDoz tablets	200
Vivarin tablets	200
Pain relievers (standard dose)	
Anacin	64
Excedrin	130
Midol	65
Plain aspirin, any brand	0
Diuretics (standard dose)	
Aqua-Ban	200
Permathene H_2Off	200
Pre-Mens Forte	100
Cold remedies (standard dose)	
Coryban-D	30
Dristan	32
Triaminicin	30
Weight-control aids (daily dose)	
Dexatrim	200
Dietac	200
Prolamine	280

[1]Copyright 1981, 1984 by Consumers Union of United States, Inc., Mount Vernon, N.Y. 10553. Adapted by permission from *Consumer Reports*, October 1981, February 1984.

Caffeine intake has not been studied to any great extent in children but some experts warn that consumption may be relatively high when expressed relative to body weight. That is, the caffeine in a cola beverage will raise the caffeine level in the blood more in a smaller person than a larger person. For adults, coffee is the largest single source of caffeine with soft drinks second. In children, soft drinks are probably the greatest source of caffeine. However, because a number of soft drinks are now caffeine-free, caffeine consumption particularly in children may now be decreasing.

People vary widely in their response to caffeine. It is estimated that the threshold quantity in adults, that is, the
amount needed to produce a stimulating effect, ranges from
150 to 250 mg. About 200 to 750 mg daily is the range considered excessive as it produces symptoms such as anxiety, restlessness, abnormal heart rhythm, diarrhea, and acid stomach.
It may not be necessary to try to eliminate all caffeine but it
would appear beneficial to reduce your consumption at times
when you are exposed to stress. Gulping three cups of coffee
an hour or two prior to an important meeting will needlessly
increase your excitability and perception of stress.

It is possible to significantly reduce your intake of caffeine
without making any dramatic changes. For example, note
from Table 13 that caffeine in coffee is strongly affected by
the manner of brewing, how long it is brewed, and whether
it is regular or instant. Some people don't like the taste of instant decaffeinated coffee but find that brewed decaffeinated
tastes more like regular brewed. Nearly all restaurants now
offer instant decaffeinated coffee and many offer brewed
decaffeinated. Until recently, caffeine was added to most soft
drinks because a beverage could not be termed a "cola" under
FDA regulations unless a certain amount of caffeine was
present. Today, a wide variety of soft drinks are available with
no caffeine whatsoever. Tea only has about one third the
caffeine of a cup of brewed coffee. By shortening the brewing
time of tea, the caffeine content can be reduced by one half
or more. Also, decaffeinated tea is available.

Many nonprescription drugs contain caffeine along with
other ingredients although there is no purpose for adding
them. There is no evidence that caffeine affects weight loss
or menstrual cramps, so most of these sources of caffeine are
worthless and could be eliminated from such drugs. It is
usually cheaper to purchase over-the-counter medications to
treat one symptom rather than a host of symptoms. Many cold
and sinus remedies, for example, include a mix of aspirin,
antihistamine, decongestant, and caffeine. Purchase them
separately and you will not only save money but you can avoid
the caffeine as well.

Because caffeine is a mildly addictive substance, when caffeine consumption decreases markedly or is eliminated in a person who normally consumes a considerable quantity, symptoms such as headache and depression can occur. These symptoms, however, are temporary.

The additive effects of caffeine are important to consider. A person ingesting caffeine from several sources could consume enough to have a real effect on getting to sleep or staying calm. Consider the following example:

1 Excedrin	130 mg
1 cup of percolated coffee	110 mg
1 Dristan	32 mg
	272 mg

Many people wouldn't bat an eyelash at taking the two pills with a cup of coffee. An intake of 272 mg will certainly have a stimulating effect and may well produce symptoms of excessive dosage such as anxiety and restlessness. Nicotine is also a stimulant and because some people often smoke as they drink coffee, it is a common means of invoking stress.

Alcohol is often mistakenly thought to be a stimulant. While the immediate effect is excitatory, its major affect is that of a depressant. Depression is a common trait in stressed people and alcohol only further adds fuel to the fire. Also, because alcohol abuse is a health problem of huge magnitude in this country, use of alcohol as a means of unwinding and seeking relief from stress is a dangerous habit.

Coping on the Move

A common question I hear from people learning stress coping techniques is that the techniques would appear to be effective when practiced in a quiet environment, but will they work in the pell-mell environment of everyday life? In other words, the techniques may help you unwind at the end of the day or when you have the time, but what can you do when stress confronts you in the workplace or at home when other people are around? Experts have several recommendations for these times when you cannot get off alone, turn off the lights, or eliminate noise or distraction. One authority suggests performing your practiced routine in your mind for 5 or 6 seconds. In other words, you visualize tensing and relaxing a group of muscles; or you could tense a smaller muscle group such as pressing the thumb and forefinger together; or you could inhale and exhale slowly once or twice. The idea is that if you have practiced the technique for weeks or months beforehand, then even a 5- or 6- second minidrill or reminder will elicit the same psychological and biological response.

Another valuable means of coping with sudden onset of stress is to employ a fitting behavior that takes the pressure off you. Some examples are given in Table 14.

Work Efficiency and Stress

The efficiency with which we do our work affects our susceptibility to stress. Scientifically speaking, efficiency is the ratio of energy expenditure to work done, so improvement of efficiency is a two-factor process. For most of us in our jobs, our energy expenditure is not a key element in our work; therefore our attention here will emphasize the amount and quality of work accomplished.

Several fundamental principles of work efficiency are commonly noted by the experts: 1) prioritize and focus your concentration on one task at a time, and 2) keep things simple. A brief explanation of each follows.

Prioritize

One of the most common errors most of us make is to do the little, easy tasks before we engage the most important ones. The "biggies" seem to encourage procrastination while

Table 14 Coping With Stress in the Real World

Event	Typical behavior	Coping behavior
Accident on freeway will make you late for work	Constantly change lanes trying to get in the one moving fastest; almost hit someone; drive aggressively and impolitely; you feel guilty about it later	Realize nothing can be done without endangering yourself or others; let a few cars into your lane and notice that it feels good to help others; react to overly aggressive drivers by shaking your head
Oversleep—will be 30 minutes late for work	Rush dressing, cut yourself shaving, tie isn't adjusted to proper length, skip breakfast	Phone office and let them know you won't be in until 9 or so; dress, shower, shave, and eat breakfast as normally do
Big exam on Friday and you want to watch a special movie on TV tonight	Watch the movie and feel guilty; lost one evening of study and start thinking negatively about the upcoming exam	Check the cable TV schedule and see that movie is to be shown twice later in the month; can see it later OR a friend with VCR agrees to tape the movie for you OR you skip aerobic dance class that afternoon OR skip regular 30 to 45 minutes of socializing; instead you get home, skim several chapters and start underlining key concepts in lecture notes;

Table 14 (Cont.)

Event	Typical behavior	Coping behavior
		study for another hour after dinner and are surprised how much you covered; you watch the movie and feel justified in doing so and therefore really enjoy it; you feel good about your initial preparation for the exam
Company tomorrow night for dinner	Panic City! Yell at the kids and husband; it's 36 hours of agony for entire household; you're semi-exhausted when company arrives and swear you won't go through this again for a long time	Organize plans on paper; switch to decaf coffee for the next 36 hours; assign husband and kids specific tasks; prepare hors d'oeuvres, table setting and guest bathroom the day before company arrives

the multiple trivial ones make us appear busy to others as well as ourselves. Therein lies much of the problem. In our society it is so "in" to appear to be superbusy. It doesn't matter what you do as long as you look busy doing it. It is a false basis of pride, however, because it places the emphasis on the process and not the product. To be productive and yet efficient, you must learn to emphasize the latter. To facilitate this, list your tasks. Rank order each of them and then get going on number 1, not numbers 8 through 11. Save an hour or two each day for maintenance type tasks such as sorting mail and making phone calls, but do them only after working for a block of time on number 1. If task number 1 is not completed by the end of the work day, make it the first thing you tackle the next day. Then, and only then, should you go on to task number 2.

I make a task list for each week and it keeps me progressing on my key objectives while letting me stay up with daily activities including meetings, phone calls, reading and sorting mail, and writing memos. Organizing your work day in this manner also facilitates scheduling things so that they interfere only minimally with the vital tasks. Many people schedule meetings or appointments only for the convenience of others. That may be admirable in a way, but it does not help their productivity. Remember that your efficiency aids your productivity because productivity is gauged by the quantity and quality of performance on the key tasks in your work. I have yet to hear of someone who received a promotion, raise or award for being an outstanding phone caller, mail reader, memo writer, or office socializer.

Keep Things Simple

This is a restatement of the famous KISS principle—*Keep It Simple, Stupid*. The major tasks we do in our work typically are somewhat complex. Therefore we need to divide them into steps in a meaningful way. Some of the steps perhaps you cannot complete at once because they may involve communication with or action by other people. This very fact discourages some people from acting on these components. However, if completion of a project hinges on this action or communication step by another person, the step should be done early in the project rather than being delayed. It is frustrating to nearly complete a project and then have to wait on someone else in order to completely finish it.

An efficient way to start any work is to list all the major components. Many people like to use an outline form while others like to draw boxes, circles, and dotted lines. All are effective. The next step is one that separates the efficient from the highly efficient. Each step needs to be related timewise to the completion of the project. Table 15 is a sample of a form I often use to indicate the status of a step or component as well as when I need to complete it.

Such a system will help guide you to the completion of a project with greater clarity of thought and greater efficiency. This system helps to identify the key components of a project,

Table 15 Timeline for Planning a Summer Vacation

Date	Action	Status (check or X when completed)
February 1	Call and reserve cabin	
March 15	Write to Triple A for pamphlets, maps, etc.	
April 21	Enroll kids in proper session of summer playground	
May 8	Register Steve for baseball Register Eric for computer class: second session	
May 15	Write or call Aunt Marge and Uncle Bill about possibly spending a night with them	

the time sequence in which each component should be accomplished, and encourages concentrating on each task by itself until it is completed. I found that it took me a project or two before the system really demonstrated its advantages. I use it for writing articles in professional publications, planning meetings, and of course, used it writing this book.

A Philosophy of Life to Reduce Stress

My comments here lack scientific evidence yet I feel sound in making them. Most of them you have heard or read before but I believe it is of value to state them here in an organized manner. Hopefully, they add a good finishing touch to this chapter. Ideally they will make your everyday worries seem smaller and more tolerable.

1.   Don't compare yourself with others. Comparisons are made too often with exceptional people; the result is almost certain to lead to a feeling of inferiority.
2.   Accept your limitations. I view diabetes as a limitation rather than a disease. The difference is the latter term to most people implies being sick, needing constant attention, and leading to a downward trend in health and function. I think such a view is so negative it stifles many diabetics. The limitations in being diabetic are small: measuring blood sugar, taking insulin or medication, adhering to consistent eating times, and in general maintaining a consistent life-style. Indeed, many of the rules for good diabetic management read like a list of health habits even millions of nondiabetics should practice to be optimally healthy.

     Mathematical probability suggests that truly outstanding human accomplishment must be something out of the ordinary. If 100,000 people had climbed Mt. Everest, the deed would become less impressive. If thousands of us could run a sub-4-minute mile, we would hardly pay much attention to people running a mile in 3 minutes and 50 seconds. The point is that even if one should strive and work endlessly over a lifetime to achieve and be noted in a given field, there simply is not room enough at the top for more than a handful of people. Realize, too, that accomplishments and talents are very specific. Is the Nobel Prize winner also an NFL star? Is he or she attractive enough to make it in Hollywood? Is he or she an active member of the PTA or church? Be realistic and achieve what you can in the most meaningful things in *your* life. Mother Nature has provided a diversity of interest and talent in a thousand different endeavors and luckily so. No one person has to be an overachiever in many facets of life, yet some people try.

3.   Create a moment of pleasure several times each day and concentrate on it while you experience the event.

Look closely at someone you love; I mean really look and study his or her features. Touch the face and listen extra carefully to this person speaking. Look into his or her eyes. Is this not a moment of pleasure?

Smile at a clerk or some other busy worker who looks hassled. Try to make that person smile. Compliment the person. Helping others and being kind to others should make you feel good.

4.   Most happiness is created and is not due to good luck.

If you view happiness in this manner, I believe it encourages seeking and creating happiness. It is all around us if we simply reach out and look. Learn to create a pleasant environment. Smile at people, say nice things, and live the Golden rule. You will find that many others are bound to do the same to you.

Summary

Stress is a common problem for most people today in our society. For the diabetic it is of particular concern because stress can raise as well as possibly lower the blood sugar level and affect the way we feel and function. A number of techniques can reduce stress including exercise, deep breathing, progressive muscle relaxation visualization, and yoga. Caffeine, nicotine, and many nonprescription drugs also can elicit or magnify the stress response and so they should be used carefully. Special techniques can be used for dealing with acute stress. Improving your work efficiency may reduce stress. Lastly, your philosophy of life is closely related to stress, and it is a force you can use to enhance your life.

chapter 11

Handling Special and Unexpected Conditions

One of the cardinal principles of diabetic management is to be as consistent as possible in eating, taking insulin or medication, and exercising. Consistency makes it easier to regulate blood sugar. However, life doesn't always allow for consistency. The purpose of this chapter is to offer suggestions regarding coping with such events as illness, eating out, traveling, surgery, and holidays. The suggestions may reduce the anxiety of doing the unusual and being jeopardized by the unexpected.

Two key guidelines that make life easier for diabetics are not to hide the fact that you are a diabetic and to use blood sugar testing as the basis for making corrections. With these essentials understood, let's take a look at how you might handle some inconsistencies of life.

Illness

Diabetics typically need more insulin or medication when they are sick because of increased secretion of the stress hormones by the adrenal gland. These hormones increase the production of glucose by the liver but reduce the uptake of glucose by the tissues. These changes tend to produce hyperglycemia and more insulin or blood sugar-lowering medication is needed to counteract this effect.

We normally reduce our physical activity when sick, increasing the need for insulin or medication. Even when nauseous, intermediate or long-acting insulin or insulin-like medication should be taken to allow normal metabolism to occur. If you are unable to eat a meal, your body will use stored fat and glycogen for energy, as well as body protein. You still need some insulin or medication, therefore, to metabolize these energy sources. For type 1 diabetics, if you are unable to eat a meal, then no rapid-acting insulin should be taken beforehand. Your intermediate or long-lasting insulin will usually cover your metabolic needs during this time. When food can be eaten, then adhere to your normal insulin schedule.

Because activity and food intake may be altered significantly and because of the tendency for adrenal hormones to raise the blood sugar, insulin dosage will have to be determined by checking blood sugar levels periodically. Some diabetologists suggest as many as seven blood sugar tests be taken daily while sick. This may necessitate several extra shots but it certainly prevents additional problems such as ketosis from occurring while one is ill. Because more insulin is needed when you are sick, be on guard for ketosis. The symptoms of your illness may somewhat mask the symptoms of ketosis and hyperglycemia, so check the urine for ketones and the blood sugar periodically.

Surgery

In a well-controlled diabetic, surgery need not be an overly complicating event. The unique concern for a diabetic during and after surgery is to maintain a reasonable level of blood sugar. For type 1 diabetics it is best to go into surgery having taken some intermediate or long-lasting insulin to prevent ketoacidosis. Since surgery is usually scheduled in the morning and you will not eat breakfast, diabetics on insulin will usually forego their regular insulin in the morning. Those with type 2 diabetes should seek the advice of their doctor regarding modification of medicine. It is best to have the blood sugar moderately elevated, perhaps 150 to 200 mg%, before surgery. This elevation will minimize the occurrence of hypoglycemia. In recovery, you should request that your blood sugar be taken to determine if glucose should be administered intravenously. You should discuss these details with your doctor. Your confidence will be greater if you know that your blood sugar level will be checked.

I have been under general anesthesia only once since I have been diabetic. I used the plan described here and had no problems whatsoever. I did my own blood sugar test at about 6:00 a.m. and purposely planned for it to be a bit high, which it was (about 180 mg%). I discussed the plan with my doctor as well as the anesthesiologist, and I felt secure because they knew my plan exactly.

Diabetics should realize that infection tends to upset blood sugar control. We require more insulin and become prone to ketoacidosis. Whether infection is the cause or result of your surgery, realize what its effect is and be prepared to do extra blood sugar tests to determine how much added insulin you may need. Any surgical procedure carries with it a slight risk of infection. Your doctor may closely check for this but you will want to carefully examine the site of surgery once you are home. Also, the emotional stress associated with hospitalization and surgery will tend to raise blood sugar. Monitor your blood sugar more frequently than normal so you can alter your diet, insulin, or medication.

Pregnancy

Until diabetics began to use insulin in the 1920s, few diabetic women became mothers. Today, well-controlled diabetics undergo minimal problems and usually deliver healthy infants. However, lack of metabolic or blood sugar control exposes both mother and fetus to complications.

As with any other erratic condition, constant attention must be paid to glucose levels and necessary adjustments made when warranted. Often, extra insulin is needed to control blood sugar, and frequently type 2 diabetics who normally regulate their condition with diet, exercise, and pills may require some insulin.

Diabetics are sometimes hospitalized in the last several weeks of pregnancy. Early deliveries are often encouraged particularly if complications appear. The fetus is typically monitored closely to ensure that oxygen supply is adequate. The diabetic mother and infant are observed closely in the days after delivery and the infant is often kept in an incubator. These procedures minimize the occurrence of complications and allow immediate intervention when necessary.

Medications

A number of medications can affect the blood sugar level in both type 1 and type 2 diabetics. Beta-blockers, used by many heart patients and people with high blood pressure, tend to lower the blood sugar. However, when a person with type 2 diabetes uses beta-blockers in combination with oral medication to control blood glucose, a drug interaction may inhibit the diabetes medication, causing an increase in blood sugar. Birth control pills tend to raise glucose levels because they inhibit insulin action and it has been found that women over age 35 on the pill have a higher incidence of cardiovascular disease. Diabetic women taking the pill will therefore need extra insulin. Because diabetes is a secondary risk factor for cardiovascular disease, some doctors prefer that their female patients use a different method of contraception.

Diuretics are commonly used by heart patients, people with high blood pressure, and people trying to lose weight. While diuretics have value for some individuals with the first two conditions, there is no advantage in fat loss because they only increase the loss of water and have no effect on fat metabolism. Important minerals are also eliminated with the water, which can make the heart beat arrhythmically and induce fatigue. Diuretics do raise the blood sugar, however. Patients who are placed on diuretics will need to carefully monitor blood sugar and determine how much extra insulin or medication is needed.

Decongestants have a slight tendency to raise the blood sugar. Prednisone, an anti-inflammatory medication, has a potent effect on blood sugar. I used it once for 3 or 4 days to aid sinus drainage and had a troublesome siege of hyperglycemia that lasted as long. I had several blood sugar tests above 300 mg% in that time. Needless to say, I haven't used prednisone since.

Note that many medications include a statement on the container or insert that diabetics should not use them unless they have been approved by a physician. The best policy for diabetics regarding medications is to present a list to your physician. He or she can then make specific recommendations.

Stress

Stress results in several hormones of the adrenal gland being secreted. Adrenaline and noradrenaline cause the liver to release glucose into the blood while cortisol inhibits the action of insulin. These effects usually cause the blood sugar to rise. However, stress is also known to cause a reduction in blood sugar at times. The key to correcting for the effect of stress is to check the blood sugar. To minimize the effects of stress one can use any number of stress-reducing strategies. Exercise not only reduces stress, but if adequate insulin is present in the blood, it also results in considerable energy expenditure, both of which will help minimize a rise in blood sugar.

If my blood sugar is elevated, I take a corrective dosage of quick-acting insulin. The dosage will depend on the blood sugar reading. When stressed or when in a stress-prone situation, it would be wise to forego caffeine and nicotine. You will be better off to use decaffeinated drinks and to stay off decongestants and medications containing caffeine.

Identification

Insulin-dependent and noninsulin-dependent diabetics should carry some readily observable identification of their condition such as a bracelet, necklace, or card in the wallet or purse. We have all heard tragic stories about hypoglycemic diabetics being jailed for drunkenness or even being mistreated or left untreated with an insulin reaction after an auto accident. Because you could be left in an unconscious state totally incapable of helping yourself, even the best-controlled diabetics should be easily identifiable. The necklace or bracelet is probably most advantageous in this regard.

Snack Food While Traveling

I always bring fresh fruit, crackers, and my homemade oatmeal cookies in my suitcase when I travel. I also put some of these items into my briefcase when I travel by air. Quite often the meal or snack served on an airplane is difficult to predict regarding its content and the time it will be served.

Fresh fruit is often unavailable in restaurants. My supplementary food supply guarantees good nutrition and I would hate to depend only on what is available in the evenings in most hotels or motels for my evening snack. Sticking with fruits and grains for snacks is cheaper and healthier, plus when you settle in for the evening, you may not want to have to dress up and leave your room again.

Emergency Supplies in the Car

Besides normal winter emergency provisions kept in a car such as sand, shovel, blankets, boots, hat and gloves, I also have a lunch box filled with dried fruit, crackers, and candy.

If I should ever be delayed in traffic or on the highway, I have my next meal plus an emergency supply of calories with me. Nearly every winter, I have spent undue time in driving home on at least one occasion due to snowy and icy driving conditions, and on several occasions I have had to use my emergency food supply. Knowing that it is there greatly reduces my anxiety when I drive in such conditions.

In my glove compartment, I have candy and a bag of dimes and quarters. Every now and then, I may be just a bit late in getting home for dinner or for some reason, symptoms of insulin reaction appear on the way home. I pop a couple of Lifesavers into my mouth after pulling over to a side street, take something from my briefcase to read, and within 5 to 10 minutes, I can safely and calmly continue driving. Again, I feel secure knowing that the candy and change are there. The change is there in case I would need to make a phone call.

Delayed Meals

I always carry one or two hard candies in my pocket or coat just in case. When going out to eat you may have to stand in a restaurant line or your host or hostess may delay dinner for some reason. If symptoms of an insulin reaction occurred, you could buy candy or a sweet drink while waiting in a restaurant and you can munch appetizers before dinner at someone's home. However, I still like to have candy on my person at all times. On airplane flights, I carry a pack of Lifesavers, snack items, and my insulin kit in my briefcase in addition to candy in my pocket. You never know.

Eating Out

Restaurant food tends to be high in fat and therefore high in calories. Diabetics and even nondiabetics can minimize calories considerably by selecting baked or broiled fish, chicken or turkey (with the skin removed). Although restaurants sometimes advertise only fried chicken or fish on the menu, they often will bake or broil it on special request. It is not an unusual or excessive request and a decent restaurant is probably quite willing to prepare your food this way.

For breakfast in a restaurant I tend to stick with oatmeal, juice, toast and coffee, or pancakes with about one third of a teaspoon of sugar on each. I don't eat eggs very often but for those who do, an eggs, toast, and juice breakfast can be ordered, which is about identical in calories and composition as the same meal cooked at home. With these simple guidelines, I feel quite comfortable eating out.

Treating Insulin Reaction

Veteran diabetics detect symptoms of hypoglycemia in its earliest stages. Symptoms include hunger, drowsiness, muscle fatigue, dizziness, muscle cramps, irritability, and elevated pulse rate. While books and articles list many possible symptoms, they do not all necessarily appear, thank goodness. Often, just one symptom becomes readily apparent. Because hunger is such a common symptom and because it can become very strong, many diabetics overeat and experience rebound hyperglycemia. Also, a drop in blood sugar causes the liver to release glucose unless excessive insulin is present in the blood. In a well-conditioned diabetic, the contribution of glucose by the liver usually prevents severe insulin reactions leading to unconsciousness. So, you needn't eat a full-fledged meal to properly treat an insulin reaction.

The goal in treating hypoglycemia is to raise the blood sugar to about 100 mg%. To do this, it is best to consume one carbohydrate exchange or about 60 calories. Before taking additional carbohydrate, the blood sugar should be checked. Most often the one carbohydrate exchange plus the glucose released by the liver will normalize the blood sugar within 15 to 20 minutes. If the blood sugar 15 to 20 minutes later is below 60 to 80 mg%, then an additional one-half carbohydrate exchange should complete the correction.

I stay away from protein and fat in treating an insulin reaction because they take too long to be digested and raise the blood sugar. Furthermore, by the time they have an effect on blood sugar, which would be about 1.5 to 3 hours later, the bout of hypoglycemia should be long over. Fats and carbohydrates, consequently, may lead to elevated blood sugar hours after an insulin reaction.

Glucagon is a pancreatic hormone that causes the blood sugar to rise by inhibiting the action of insulin and increasing the release of glucose from the liver. It can be injected like insulin into a diabetic who is unconscious or semiconscious due to insulin reaction. Family and close friends should be taught to administer an injection of glucagon.

Treating an Insulin Reaction in Public

This was a tough nut for me to crack for many years. I was always afraid of being discovered as a diabetic, and until I was nearly 30 years old, I hid the fact. I can remember several bad experiences created from my insecurity. On one occasion in college, I was umpiring a softball game. The symptoms of hypoglycemia slowly crept over me and I didn't have my usual candy in my pocket. Rather than calling time-out and going to my car to get candy, I stuck it out to the end of the game. Calling balls and strikes while seeing two balls and sweating copiously isn't easy, and I shun to think of the bad calls I must have made. It was unfair to the ball players and unfair to jeopardize myself like that. Please don't do that to yourself. Be honest with people and let them know what is happening. Few people are going to mind a brief interruption particularly if they know the reason.

Ever since I was able to break the ice and tell people I was diabetic if such was appropriate, I have saved myself at lot of anxiety. Today if I should ever need to pull out my Lifesavers in public I do not hesitate. It is not uncommon for someone to suck on a candy during a meeting or in many other situations, so attention to such an action is probably minimal anyway.

I once addressed a group of diabetics at 11:00 a.m. and while walking into the hospital where the meeting was held, noticed I was beginning to go into insulin reaction. I strolled into the meeting with two Lifesavers in my mouth and asked for a glass of orange juice, which was available in the back of the room. I sipped my juice and introduced myself as their speaker, an insulin-dependent diabetic having an insulin reaction. I asked for a brief respite and then gave my talk. We had a good laugh at my having a reaction before talking to them, but it was probably instructive for them as well.

Treating Ketoacidosis

Ketones are by-products of normal fat metabolism and so are produced in nondiabetics and diabetics. Fat breakdown is exaggerated, however, when insufficient insulin is present in the blood to allow the normal utilization of glucose in the tissues. Ketosis, then, occurs when an excessive quantity of ketone bodies, which are strong acids, accumulate in the blood. The term ketoacidosis is synonymous with ketosis but adds the descriptive term "acid."

Ketoacidosis occurs if insulin is not administered, if the dosage of insulin administered is inadequate, or if an unusually stressing event such as an injury, shock, anxiety, or infection occurs. It rarely occurs in type 2 diabetics. When such situations do happen, extra blood sugar tests should be done. If the blood sugar reaches 300 mg% or higher, the urine should be checked for ketones. Before insulin was discovered, many diabetic adults and most diabetic children eventually went into coma and died from this condition.

The symptoms of ketoacidosis are excess urination, nausea, vomiting, abdominal pain, dry skin, shortness of breath, fruity odor of the breath, elevated pulse rate, and finally unconsciousness. These symptoms can appear quite suddenly in type 1 diabetics but take several days to appear in type 2 diabetics. To treat this condition, large and/or frequent doses of regular insulin are given in an attempt to lower the blood sugar and enhance the utilization of glucose in the cells. Once the breakdown of glucose and fat is returned to a normal rate, ketone production will also drop to normal. Fluid replacement is critical to minimize the relative concentrations of the strongly acidic ketones in the blood.

You should definitely develop a plan regarding ketosis with your physician. Most physicians would want to be contacted immediately if ketones are found in the urine. If the blood sugar can be quickly stabilized with additional regular insulin, hospitalization may not be necessary. However, understand that the treatment may necessitate giving fluids intravenously and constantly monitoring blood glucose and ketone levels. If you are at the stage where you are nauseous or vomiting, and can't consume fluid and conduct these tests at home, you certainly should be hospitalized.

The best policy regarding ketosis is prevention. Know when it is likely to occur, and check your blood sugar and ketone levels. Ketosis is a dangerous state that can be largely avoided by adequate management.

Prolonged Inactivity

Prolonged physical inactivity should be an unusual situation for a diabetic actively taking charge of his or her condition. On days of relative inactivity either more insulin should be taken to cover the energy not expended in exercise or less food should be eaten. However, I don't know of many diabetics who are willing to eat less than they are accustomed to eating.

I usually take extra insulin on days that I drive or fly for more than an hour or two. However, if the travel is done in the afternoon and evening, I can get by without extra insulin if I get an extra hard or long workout in during the morning. If I need the extra insulin, I know that an extra 2 units of regular insulin before dinner will be needed if the travel time is about 4 to 6 hours. If I can't exercise during the day and sit virtually the whole day, I take 2 extra units of lente in the morning for long-term coverage of my relative inactivity and 1 extra unit of regular before lunch. I check my blood sugar before dinner to see how things balanced out during the day and take extra regular insulin if needed. If the family is with me, I normally jog and/or swim in a motel pool with my sons in the early evening. It has also become a habit of ours to always keep ball gloves in the car and to toss for awhile after lunch when we're on the road traveling. Boy, does that feel good after sitting all morning!

Those with type 2 diabetes can also increase the amount of oral medication taken when less physically active than normal, but you should do so only under the advice of your physician. Excessive medication could lead to insulin reaction.

Prolonged Physical Activity

When prolonged physical activity such as backpacking, working in the yard, spring cleaning, or running a marathon is undertaken, a reduction in insulin or oral medication is usually required to prevent insulin reaction. I was able to run a marathon (26.2 miles) several years ago quite comfortably without any episodes of hypoglycemia. Whereas I normally took 4 units of regular insulin and 12 units of lente in the morning, I reduced my regular insulin to just 1 unit and made no change in my lente insulin. I then had a normal breakfast of cereal, juice, and tea. The overall reduction in insulin was not great for several reasons. First, I had been able to do my daily training run each day in the early morning for the 6 or 7 weeks preceding the marathon. I did this because the event was to start at 6:00 a.m. to avoid the August heat in the middle of the day. By training in the morning about an hour after breakfast each day, I was able to avoid extreme temperatures. Second, the same amount of insulin taken in the morning has a lesser blood sugar-lowering effect than if taken later in the day. Thus, it is usually better for me to do prolonged exercise in the morning. Note that I didn't even have to decrease my lente insulin because it wouldn't have any effect on my blood sugar until well after the marathon was completed. Third, each Sunday morning for nearly 4 months before the marathon, I did my single longest run of each week. Starting at about 10 miles, I gradually progressed to 23 miles. So, I knew pretty well how much my daily insulin would have to be altered for running hours at a time. Consequently, by race day, my insulin, water, and sugar intake formula had been tested repeatedly.

I drank a good amount of water and Gatorade at the aid stations, which were spaced every 3 miles. I mixed water and Gatorade about half and half so that it wasn't very concentrated. Dilution of sweet or salty beverages allows water to pass more quickly from the stomach and intestine into the blood. So, because of the heat and threat of dehydration my first concern was water and only secondarily was I concerned about low blood sugar.

Once again, I knew from my daily training runs and particularly from the long run on Sundays how long I could exert before being prone to hypoglycemia. Endurance training in diabetics as well as nondiabetics greatly increases the time one can exercise or work before most of the muscle and liver glycogen are depleted. In an untrained person this may happen in 45 to 60 minutes, whereas in trained people it seems to take 2.5 to well over 3 hours. When these tissues become depleted of glycogen, the exerciser becomes unduly fatigued and slows his or her work pace to a crawl or stops to eat. Marathon runners, however, do not wish to stop to eat, so they sometimes resort to consuming some carbohydrate while they run or as they stop momentarily every 3 miles at an aid station, where they consume water and diluted fruit juice, cola, or other beverages or snacks.

A second major advantage to prolonging the point of exhaustion is that endurance-trained muscles metabolize fat to a greater extent than untrained muscles. This reduces the breakdown of muscle glycogen with the result that the time of exercise can be extended. It is believed that the extra-long running session performed weekly by most marathoners greatly enhances their capacity to metabolize fat. When exercise lasts beyond about 30 minutes, certain hormones accelerate the breakdown of fat in our fat deposits. These fats are released into the blood and eventually are delivered to the working muscles. The better trained the muscles are for long work, the more readily they use these fats for fuel.

So, my muscles were quite well-trained for long work as I averaged about 52 miles per week of running over the last 10 weeks before the marathon. I did start to use a squeeze tube of honey at 16 miles. I held it in my hand while running and took about a dozen sucks from it the last 10 miles. I think I used it primarily for security just in case I began to sense hypoglycemia, but the symptoms never appeared. By the 24th mile nothing could have stopped me and my sense of elation at this point made me realize I could probably go beyond 26.2 miles if necessary. I finished with a "kick," having averaged 8 minutes and 54 seconds per mile. Hardly a fast pace but it represented meeting a challenge common to many runners. It also demonstrated to me that well-controlled diabetics can participate in arduous, prolonged exercise. The diabetic who completed the notorious Ironman Triathlon in Hawaii is also strong supporting evidence for this contention.

I have learned to use small, frequent snacks when I backpack in the Colorado Rockies every summer. Because most of my hikes begin in the early morning, I reduce my morning regular insulin by 1 or 2 units if my blood sugar is 130 mg% or less. I eat one or two extra carbohydrate exchanges and one extra protein exchange. By the time I hit the trail, usually about 45 minutes after breakfast, I am burning some of the carbohydrate from my breakfast and by middle or late morning my breakfast protein probably begins to supply some of my energy.

For my morning hikes I use the same amount of lente insulin when backpacking as I do at home. This may sound surprising but I am also physically active enough at home in the summer that the difference in energy expenditure isn't terribly great. Several summers ago I estimated the calories expended while backpacking each day based on my heart rate. In my laboratory at the university I had previously determined how many calories I expended at a number of different heart rates while walking and jogging on a treadmill. (This was done by measuring the amount of oxygen I consumed each minute. Oxygen consumption can be converted to caloric expenditure.) This allowed me to convert heart rate to calories while backpacking. I averaged expending about 1200 calories backpacking in the mountains each day. Most of the hikes lasted 3 to 4 hours while one lasted 6 hours and took me to 13,000 feet elevation. The caloric cost of that backpacking session was nearly 2,000 calories.

I also measured my blood sugar four times daily. Figure 13 summarizes my blood sugar readings for the week in the mountains and for the previous week at home teaching, jogging, working in the yard, playing ball with my boys, and other activities. The average blood sugars at home at 7:00 a.m.,

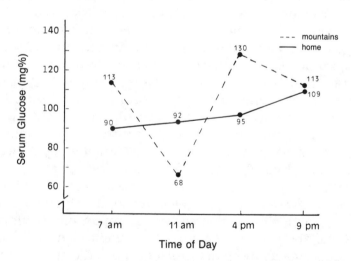

Figure 13   Blood glucose data during 6 days of backpacking and 6 days at home (With permission, from Berg, K.E., 1983. Blood glucose regulation in an insulin-dependent diabetic backpacker. *The Physician and Sportsmedicine*, **11**[12], 103.)

11:00 a.m., 4:00 p.m., and 9:00 p.m. ranged from 90 to 109 mg%. This represents a high degree of control. In the mountains the blood sugar averaged from 68 to 130 mg%. These scores also indicate good control according to several current publications in the medical literature. The average of 68 mg% occurred at 11:00 a.m. and reflects the energy expended in several hours of backpacking each morning. I had only one occasion where symptoms of hypoglycemia occurred and this was minor and quickly handled by consuming dried fruit and granola. The low values at 11:00 a.m. suggest I could have reduced my morning regular insulin another unit, I could have consumed more fruit and granola periodically while hiking, or I could have eaten additional protein for breakfast.

Some authorities recommend eating carbohydrate (one exchange) every 20 to 30 minutes during prolonged exercise. I have never had to consume food at this rate but I think it has something to do with a person's training level. More highly trained people will be able to use fat as an energy source to a greater extent than lesser-trained individuals, and their muscles and liver store more glycogen. So, glycogen depletion and insulin reaction will be less likely to occur in trained diabetics.

If exercise is to continue much into the afternoon, the dosage of intermediate or long-lasting insulin should probably be reduced. One authority suggests a reduction of 50% of the normal dosage of intermediate or long-acting insulin when exercise lasts all day. I have found this to be a bit extreme for me but again it may be a result of being quite physically active. In the medical literature, some diabetics exercising all day are able to reduce their insulin by 75% and still not suffer hypoglycemia or ketosis. As with so many facets of diabetic management, I think the guidelines are a good starting point. However, everyone will respond differently to the same regimen, which underscores the importance of individualizing diabetic management. The key to individualizing is blood sugar measurement, so do extra blood tests when you are unusually active and bring your equipment with you when you head off into the wilderness.

Whenever I head out for exercise that is to last longer than normal, I carry a pack of Lifesavers and a quarter. I rarely have insulin reactions, but about twice a year I will develop symptoms while exercising. Once I pulled a muscle stumbling over a bush while running. I was about 6 miles from home and I did have my emergency pack, that is, my candy and quarter. I didn't need to use the candy but I did use the quarter to phone my wife to pick me up. You will feel more secure on long treks with those items along, which should enhance the enjoyment of the exercise.

On the Job

I keep snack foods, emergency candy, insulin, and supplies for blood sugar testing in my office. I don't often check my blood during the day, but at times when I feel tired, irritable or just plain "funny," it's good to know I can do a quick check and take corrective action with food or insulin. At the office I do my blood sugar testing without my glucometer but instead rely on the color comparison technique.

We get occasional blizzards and ice storms in Omaha. Although it has never happened, if I should ever not be able to make it home, I have my insulin and am ready.

Staying on Schedule With Insulin and Oral Medication

This is a sacred principle for good diabetic control because eating, exercise, and everything else seems to depend on having this variable be as constant as possible. I set my alarm for 6:30 a.m. and never deviate if I can possibly help it. If you don't get up at the same time each day to take your insulin or medication, then attaining and maintaining good blood sugar control is going to be far more complex, and for many, impossible. So, get up every day at the same time to take your insulin or medication and take your insulin at the same time of day if you take several injections.

It is awkward and inconvenient at times to get up and leave a meeting, seek privacy, and take your shot. I rarely take my insulin in front of anyone but this is my own limitation. A young 8-year-old friend of my youngest son has insulin-dependent diabetes. At my son's last birthday party, his friend brought his insulin kit and administered his shot in front of several of the youngsters. The children observing were interested and several made comments like, "Atta way, Mark!" or "Hey, that's neat, Mark!" I thought it was pretty neat too, particularly his doing it in front of the others.

Even if you don't wish to take insulin in public, at least be willing to excuse yourself from a meeting, class, ballgame, party, or whatever to "stick" to your schedule. It makes life so much easier.

I usually resort to using a restroom or bathroom to administer my insulin. I often feel like Superman searching for a phone booth.

Holidays

Holidays are a good test of a diabetic's overall skills, knowledge, and discipline. It's only natural to want to enjoy special treats and partake of good times in general. Artificial sweeteners are used by many diabetics and nondiabetics alike, so making low calorie special desserts will be attractive for many people. Dietetic candies and low-cal beverages allow diabetics to have desserts and sweets and yet adhere to sound dietary guidelines. However, nearly everyone will consume more calories for at least one special meal. For a Thanksgiving or Christmas dinner or for a picnic at the family reunion, I advise being realistic. Know yourself and if you know you are going to eat more food than usual, take some extra regular insulin about 45 minutes before the meal. You will need to take enough insulin to cover the extra food and you will certainly want to do a blood check about 2 hours afterward to see how well things are balanced. If you ate extra protein and fat as well as extra carbohydrate, realize that the effect on your blood sugar from protein and fat will not occur for several hours. So, I would recommend checking the blood sugar about 2 hours after eating to see if the regular insulin adequately covered the extra carbohydrate. An hour or two later, do another blood sugar test to see if the extra insulin was adequate to handle the protein and fat content of the meal. If you have type 2 diabetes, ask your doctor how you can adjust to such times. Many physicians are willing to make special allowances if the patient normally maintains good blood sugar control.

Unless you are willing to do several extra blood sugar tests, I would not recommend the above procedure. As you may know, the best and easiest way to maintain good regulation of blood sugar is not to lose control in the first place. In addition, I would use this plan of adding insulin for extra eating at only one meal or feeding. If you try to eat beyond your normal level for every meal and snack, then even the best-regulated diabetic will find it extremely difficult to maintain good control. If you become hyperglycemic, you certainly won't feel good emotionally, which will dampen your enjoyment of the occasion.

During the holidays, other facets of your lifestyle may be prone to change such as getting up later in the morning or not exercising. Without question, the best plan is to do as you normally do. Do take your morning insulin or pill at the same time and do your regular exercise. Things in general tend to change during holidays and the wise diabetic will keep the basics of control (such as insulin, diet, and exercise) as constant as possible.

chapter 12

Motivation

This is the most important chapter in this book for without the necessary motivation you will not actually use the information. Because my goal in writing this book is to help others with diabetes, please pay particularly close attention to this chapter. You may wish to refer to it periodically as you strive to become a healthier person.

As a former athlete and coach, and as a teacher, I have always been fascinated with what motivates people. I have studied the topic carefully because it relates so closely to my effectiveness as a teacher as well as my own life. First of all, realize that the information in this book is meant to affect your lifestyle. Lifestyle implies behavior and habits over a lifetime. Unless you view this book as a vehicle for long-term change, you stand little chance of experiencing any significant effects. The benefits of exercise, sound nutrition, and good diabetic management cannot be stored. The benefits are only provided as long as the appropriate behavior is used. Diabetics in particular, but also nondiabetics, must bank on the average health habits used over a lifetime. This is the premise of modern diabetic management.

In order to effect changes in health habits, experts recommend analyzing your present health behavior. By understanding your present eating habits, for example, you can determine exactly what changes should be made regarding your diet. The compiling of data with a plan for changing specific facets of your habits is called behavior modification. Detailed suggestions to modify behavior appear later in this chapter. Prior to looking at specific changes, it should be helpful to examine your health behavior in a more general way.

The renowned psychologist Maslow developed a model of human behavior that held that people have a hierarchy of needs to fulfill. The first and most basic need is providing the biological requirements of life such as obtaining food, shelter, and clothing. As one's basic needs are met, higher order needs must be achieved in order for a person to function adequately in society. Self-actualization is the need for which Maslow has become so well-known because it seems to be the one on which most people in the Western World focus their attention. The more basic needs of most Americans are satisfied to a reasonable extent, and consequently we spend a large part of our energy attempting to achieve higher order needs such as self-actualization. Self-actualization is the process of reaching your potential. To a diabetic, achieving good control of blood sugar should be viewed as a biological need, yet it is closely related to reaching a reasonable level of self-actualization. Therefore, for diabetics, so much of what we can become and how we function each day are largely determined by the degree we maintain good diabetic control. Your resolve, then, in monitoring your blood sugar, eating properly, and exercising regularly should be greatly strengthened.

Principles of Motivation

One of the most meaningful presentations on becoming motivated I ever heard or read was a presentation given by the head football coach at Rice University, Homer Rice. I don't think his approach contains any one novel idea, but I do believe his system has great potential because it systematizes motivation and allows it to be an active process. It is more than simply wishing hard that you can do something. Here is a summary of his motivation plan.

1. *You must really want to do something in order to be motivated.*

To focus on a particular goal, write it down so what you wish to achieve becomes clear. Second, set a date for achieving the goal, and third, write out a detailed plan of action indicating what you will do to achieve it. Last, set aside a few minutes each day to visualize having achieved the goal. Table 16 provides a step-by-step example. For this example, I have chosen a diabetic whose goal is to achieve better control over blood glucose, a goal common to all diabetics.

Table 16   Summary of Steps for Achieving a Goal

1.	Goal	To achieve better regulation of blood sugar; specifically that in the next 30 days only 2 blood sugar tests will be over 200 mg% and only 5 will be 151 to 199 mg%. All others will be 150 mg% or less.
2.	Target Date	May 1 to May 31.
3.	Plan of Action	•Measure glucose 3 times daily: before breakfast, before dinner, and before retiring.
		•Maintain tighter control over calories consumed at each feeding. Start measuring food amounts so a fairly exact count of calories can be made.
		•On days I don't exercise, administer X units of regular insulin at the time I would normally be exercising.
		•Each evening before dinner get off alone and for 60 seconds, close eyes and visualize how good I will feel mentally and physically after having achieved this goal.
		•Visualize the hemoglobin in your blood to be cleaner and unencumbered by glucose: See its enhanced ability to dump more oxygen into your tissues. Envision an enhanced oxygen supply to your muscles, kidneys, retina, and other body parts. Note that you feel better all over with this improved oxygenation to all the cells of your body.

2. *Have faith in your ability to achieve your goals.*
       Obviously the goal has to be realistic if you are to really believe you can accomplish it. Don't shoot for the impossible. By stating your goal in specific, behavioral terms and by visualizing your achievement of it you are well ahead of most people's desires to be successful. Believe in yourself and program yourself for success.
3. *Learn to be decisive.*
       Most people change their goals constantly or they limit themselves by looking at short-term goals only. Consequently, they make decisions based on a limited perspective or view of their lives. Having well-thought-out goals, a plan of attack, and a deadline should allow you to make decisions more quickly and more soundly because you know what you are striving to achieve. All decisions and actions you make thereafter can be related to the consequences they may have on these priority goals. Achievers, after carefully thinking about their goals, will be able to act more decisively and should find that they change their minds less often. Nonachievers will always have problems making decisions because they don't have a clear idea of where they are headed and so they are unsure as to the effects of ongoing decisions they must make.
       Most of us often find that our inability to decide what to do about a certain thing is more frustrating than the actual act of doing something once we have decided. Such a state is a real time-waster as well as source of frustration.
4. *Use the subconscious mind.*
       The conscious mind, as Homer Rice explains, collects all the experiences we accumulate over a lifetime, whereas the unconscious part of our mind causes us to perform or act. Our subconscious continually affects our thoughts, feelings, and actions. It is a potent force that provides a sense of intuition; it integrates all of our experiences and provides the basis for all thought, word, and action. Use of the subconscious part of your mind only requires that you repetitively, consistently, and daily

visualize yourself being successful in the specific activity you have set as your goal. Over a period, your conscious mind believes that you have actually done the very thing that is your goal. The conscious mind cannot distinguish between fact and fiction, that is, between visualization and reality. To the conscious brain, visualization is a reality.

Scientific support for this phenomenon does exist. A team of researchers in a study measured the effect of visualization, or what some people in sports call mental practice, on shooting free throws in basketball. Two groups practiced shooting for identical periods and number of days per week, but one of the two groups visualized successful shooting several minutes each day in addition to their free throw shooting. Both groups were shooting more accurately at the end of several weeks but the latter group experienced significantly more progress than the group that only did the physical practice.

Realize that visualization seems to work more effectively if you actually envision the successful act rather than merely doing the physical act. It is common in competitive sport for athletes to perform mental practice on a regular basis. A point to emphasize here is that visualization can probably be equally effective in all aspects of life. If you are going to make a speech or take on a new job responsibility, the technique should be helpful. As the days of successful imagery pass, you probably will note less anxiety and inhibition when you actually perform the activity in practice or on the job. There are most likely many reasons why visualization should enhance performance.

To many people it may seem too simple to have any dramatic effect. To be a believer, however, you must try it and experience it. I would suggest trying visualization for just one aspect of your life. Stick with it for 30 days and make sure you practice every single day. Imagine every detail of yourself successfully performing the activity: Create a slow motion film in your mind and play it back to study the detail. Perceive how it feels psychologically: If it is a physical task, feel the action in your muscles. Hear the roar of the crowd; envision yourself as a champion!

If it works, then stick with it so that the perception and memory remain firmly entrenched in your mind. After experiencing initial success with the technique, apply it to a second high priority goal as well. Learning to program your mind for success could represent a turning point in your life. It's exciting just to think of its potential.

Analysis of Factors That Affect Behavior

Social scientists gain an understanding of human behavior, both group as well as individual, by listing all the forces that exert an effect on the person, persons, group, or institution involved. They categorize each force as to whether it has a positive or negative effect on a specific behavior or group of behaviors. This systematic analysis attempts to provide a better understanding of why people act in certain ways. You and I can do the same to understand what forces may affect us in terms of our health habits. What forces increase and decrease the tendency to eat inappropriately? What forces affect our sleep, exercise habits, drinking habits? The analysis itself doesn't create improved health habits, but it can be a first step to sorting out and identifying key forces that affect us. If combined with appropriate motivational techniques such as those previously discussed, it becomes a meaningful tool to a better way of life. Table 17 summarizes an analysis of factors that might affect a person's likelihood of starting and maintaining a fitness program. Listing the positive and negative forces allows you to see where you might make changes to facilitate practicing a good health habit. A discussion with the family about starting an exercise program could produce

Table 17 Analysis of Factors Affecting a Person's Exercise Habits

Factors	Positive	Negative	Possible Action
Family	1. They love me and will support anything that is potentially good for me. 2. It would be good for my husband and children to be together a while without my being there.	1. Exercise may mean my husband will have to babysit several times a week.	1. Ask my husband and kids to join me once or twice a week. The kids could ride their bicycles while we walk.
Job	1. Exercise may help my back and make standing less painful.	1. No problems here.	
Spouse	1. He would probably be happy if I lost some weight. 2. This may help him become more fit and lose weight: He needs it.	1. He may complain at first.	1. Have him join me

(Cont.)

Table 17 (Cont.)

Factors	Positive	Negative	Possible Action
Children	1. The kids would love bicycling with us. 2. It would be good for the kids to be alone with my husband occasionally. 3. The bicycling would be good for the kids, especially Tommy.	1. The kids will probably complain the first time I go off without them.	1. I will explain to the children why I need the exercise.
Time	1. I really do have the time; I collapse after dinner and cleaning the kitchen but I really think some exercise would perk me up in the evening.		
Friends	1. Sally or June would probably like to join me whenever possible; we've talked about this the last several years but just haven't done it.		1. Call Sally and June tomorrow.

compromises between a husband and wife in caring for the children. Your four weekly jogging sessions might be traded for several blocks of time for your spouse to do something while you spend time with the children, or you might make one or two of the exercise sessions each week a family outing. The kids could bicycle or kick a soccer ball in the park while you and your spouse walk. The idea behind this analysis is to simply write things down so that you can focus at least on one critical factor to make it easier for you to change. Writing forces us to think and prioritize, and it provides hope and enthusiasm. People who take a few minutes to plan like this find that it stimulates action and a positive attitude.

The Ascending Health Spiral

A phenomenon that I have consistently noticed in people who undertake positive changes in their health habits is the improvement in their attitude regarding other health habits. In short, creation of one good habit seems to stimulate development of other good habits. I call this the ascending health spiral. In part, it may be that people who feel better physically wish to do more to feel even better. It may also provide a sense of mastery or achievement, which makes attaining other goals more challenging. As self-confidence and self-concept grow, the desire and willingness to be better probably grow along with it.

I mention this because it should be a force that is going to help you after your initial successes. In effect, you become increasingly capable of making changes, which in turn raises your psychological powers. So, the results of improving health are not merely additive in the typical sense but they often appear to be exponential. After achieving a month of good glucose control or a month of consistent exercise, you may possess a measure of motivation and self-discipline in health habits several times stronger than ever before. For these reasons, I often tell a person that the best way to begin a personal health improvement program is by mastering one facet of health behavior. For example, after doing 30 minutes of aerobic exercise consistently for several months, you may find that you just can't continue smoking or drinking excessively any longer. The one habit steamrolls you into making other positive changes. Once you have mastered your initial health goal you are a force to be reckoned with.

A Theory of Health Behavior

For decades, health educators have sought to explain why some people practice sound health behaviors while others seemingly live in denial of recognizing sound health information. Behavior is certainly a complex matter. However, one currently popular theory attempts to explain health behavior. The theory is called the Health Belief Model and very briefly it holds that people either believe that they are in control of their health, that is, their actions affect their health, or that their actions do not affect their health. The first group has what is called an internal locus of control and they attempt to modify their lives to achieve better control. These people, in theory, should be prone to taking up exercise, changing their diets, and if they are diabetics, strictly monitoring and controlling their blood sugar levels. The second group has an external locus of control and obviously they are going to be resistant to changing lifestyle.

The theory may provide insight regarding health behavior. For example, those who do not regularly exercise predominantly cite factors they are unable to control in explaining why they don't exercise, such as lack of time, poor weather, and lack of interest. This theory appears to be a relatively good basis for understanding why even scientific facts by the truckload will not by themselves change some people's behavior. The theory suggests that people with an external locus of control should focus on the perceived barriers to health change such as lack of time and lack of interest. These people might be able to find the time and interest if they were counselled on time management, for example, or if they were informed as to exactly how glucose control reduces diabetic complications. It would seem that the locus of control should first be determined, and then appropriate steps made that are particularly suited to that type of control.

At this point, I recommend to the reader to determine if your locus of control is internal or external. If it is internal, glancing once a week at chapter 2 regarding the benefits of good diabetic control may be a strong motivating force. If you are external, then consider the suggestions in the previous paragraph.

Tips on Eating for Weight Control

The chapter on weight control (chapter 9) explained in some detail several recommendations for preparing food and several theories on appetite and satiety, and summarized the calorie content of various foods. This may be a good time to review some of these concepts. Here, recommendations are made regarding motivational aspects of eating such as the buying, storing, and serving of food, and eating habits.

Storing Food

Visually display your goal on the refrigerator. If you confront your goal every time you approach the refrigerator, you may be motivated not to overeat and not to eat unless you really should.

Don't keep junk foods on hand. A day's worth of self-control may momentarily wane as you think of the ice cream in the freezer or the Twinkies in the cupboard. It is acceptable for diabetics to occasionally have a dessert item in their meal plan if they make allowance for it. It may be far easier, however, to leave the house to get an ice cream cone rather than having a whole half-gallon in the freezer tantalizing you all evening. It's too easy to cheat in a moment of weakness when such items are around. Most of us are not as likely to lose control and "pig out" with foods such as an apple, banana, sandwich, or bowl of cereal. Oh, yes, don't keep the junk foods around for unexpected guests or "for the kids." It will be easier on you if you buy exactly what is needed and use it immediately. Toss the remainder away and you can relax knowing "it" won't be around to taunt you.

Reduce the number of visual cues in your refrigerator. Are you guilty of opening the refrigerator door and "window shopping?" Cover leftovers with aluminum foil to make window shopping less interesting.

Serving Food

Use a small plate. Serve food on a smaller plate to make the quantity appear larger.

Serve filling foods and beverages. Drink fluid before and with each meal to speed up feeling full. Serve soup frequently for the same reason. One study demonstrated that 60 fewer calories were consumed when soup was added to meals. Serve bulky foods such as vegetables, breads, and fruits. These foods are high in nutritional density (i.e., nutrient value per ounce of serving) and relatively low in calories because they are mostly low in fat, and they are filling.

Don't cook more than what is needed. You will be tempted to overeat just to avoid having leftovers.

Eating

Eat slowly. Make eating an enjoyable time to socialize with family or friends. Allow time for the chemical regulators of appetite and satiety to work. Put your spoon or fork on the plate during the meal and concentrate on conversation periodically.

Give up your membership to the clean plate club. Leave a small portion of food on your plate at each meal simply to demonstrate control over your eating. Cleaning the plate of the last morsel of food may suggest to your subconscious that you finished the meal still hungry. Leaving a bite or two may convince your subconscious that you are pleasantly full and that you do not require the last bite or any other additional food.

Leave the kitchen. After you have eaten, clean up and get out. Do not nibble on leftovers. Exit stage left and get busy with something to get your mind off food. Realize that you may not feel satisfied right away because it usually takes about 30 minutes for your blood sugar level to rise after eating.

Be wary of eating while watching TV or reading. It is too easy to overeat while watching TV, studying, or reading. For one thing, we are less aware of how much we are actually eating. A bowl of popcorn may suddenly appear to have emptied itself and we look at the bowl as if to say "Who stole some of my popcorn?" I realize it's part of our culture to eat while we sit and watch TV, so I would at least urge you to take your planned allotment of a TV snack and once it is gone let it be gone. It is too easy to think that one more little helping won't hurt, but such a view may make good blood sugar control and weight control impossible. It is much easier if you dispense with the "master bowl of popcorn" philosophy in which a monstrous bowl or sack is present so that everyone can refill his or her bowl at will. If someone needs a refill, let them return to the kitchen for it.

Control the evening snack. Most diabetics are allotted an evening snack. As discussed in the chapter on weight control, there is a disadvantage in consuming a lot of calories in the evening hours; more fat is formed and the blood cholesterol level is raised. For these reasons, it is best not to consume a large snack if you need to lose weight or if your cholesterol level is too high. For others, the number of calories taken in the evening can be manipulated by taking a bit more insulin, which has its peak effect during the evening or while you are asleep. Lean diabetics can get by with having a larger evening snack as long as it is balanced with enough insulin or medication to result in a near normal blood sugar reading in the morning.

Don't let a single break in diet lead to a binge. Every diabetic has occasional slips in discipline but I think it is far preferable to give yourself some leeway for being human and not to crash emotionally. What works reasonably well for me is to take some extra regular insulin if I err. I inject into the triceps muscle on the back of the arm and then do two or three sets of push-ups, which increases the absorption of the injected insulin. This keeps my blood sugar from going sky-high. A follow-up blood sugar check several hours later lets me know if I administered enough insulin.

Assess your diet occasionally. Record everything you eat and drink for several days including a Saturday or Sunday. If you have a home computer, you can purchase inexpensive software that will do a detailed nutritional analysis. The report provides information on vitamins, minerals, protein, fat, and calories. Many universities and hospitals do these assessments for a minimal fee. The results often surprise people, including diabetics. It's easy to stray from a healthy diet, and the results from a nutritional analysis can be motivating to eat in a more controlled fashion.

Allow yourself an occasional dessert. Even diabetics can have an occasional sweet if it is accounted for. A limited quantity of sweets when taken at the end of a meal does not cause an overly rapid rise of blood sugar, so it may be preferable to have the sweet at the end of a meal rather than as a snack.

Buying Food

Don't shop when hungry. I think we have all experienced the effects of how undisciplined our food buying can become when we are hungry. The axiom here is to shop soon after you have eaten.

Shop only from a list. Make out your shopping list an hour after you have eaten when your stomach is full and your discipline regarding food is high.

Avoid the inner aisles. The primary nutrients in grocery stores such as produce, meats, poultry and fish, and dairy products are usually located in the outside aisles. Avoid the inner aisles where the junk foods tend to be located unless you have need of a specific item.

If it's not there, it can't be eaten. Berg's Law of Food Accessibility suggests that if you never buy the Twinkies, cookies, or candy, you are less likely to eat them. The American habit of spending the evening in front of the television makes us very vulnerable to sweets, chips, and ice cream during the evening. I think a better way to satisfy a craving for sweets is to eat them occasionally but out of the house. In a restaurant you may be less likely to splurge uncontrollably and inhale half a box of cookies or a half-gallon of ice cream.

Eating Out

Make special requests. If you don't want a food item that comes with a meal, tell the waiter or waitress not to bring it. If you wish the bread or rolls to be taken away after having your allotment, request it. Don't be afraid to ask if the chef can specially prepare your food even if it is not on the menu. For example, ask if you can have your chicken or fish baked or broiled rather than fried; request milk instead of cream for your coffee. Take charge and try to get what is best for you. You usually pay the same price for it either way.

Helping Children

A recent study demonstrated that parents can play a critical role in helping children lose weight. Children 8 to 12 years old were randomly placed into one of three groups. In one group obese parents and their obese children together used a special diet plan to attempt to lose weight. Foods were classified by color with red being high caloric items, yellow was foods of intermediate caloric value, and green represented low-calorie foods. In a second group, children but not their parents used the special diet. In a third group, children and parents were encouraged to lose weight but used no special diet plan.

While all three groups lost similar amounts of weight initially, the combined parent-children group using the special color-coded diet plan was significantly leaner 5 years later. Forty percent of the children in this group achieved and maintained normal weight over the 5-year period. Interestingly, children who dieted alone were more obese 5 years later as were those children not using any special diet plan. The results suggest that the combination of behavioral modification and parental support is important in children's maintaining weight loss.

Tips on Developing an Exercise Habit

Polls and surveys typically include the following reasons for people not exercising:

1. I'm too busy; no time.
2. Everyday activity keeps me fit.
3. Fitness is a fad.
4. Excessive exercise may enlarge the heart, which will be harmful when I stop exercising.
5. Occasional walking is enough for the elderly and middle-aged.
6. Exercise builds up the appetite and causes over-eating.
7. Controlling how much I eat is more important than exercise.
8. I'm too lazy.
9. Housework keeps me busy.
10. I have health problems.
11. Exercise is boring.
12. I am too old.
13. Exercise tires me.

The point to be made in listing reasons why people do not exercise is to analyze what seems to be their common theme. Nearly all portray a passive attitude about life, whereas some are simply wrong. (Note to the reader: Can you identify the ones that are scientifically invalid? Refer to chapter 3 on the benefits of exercise if you need help.) To make a significant change in your life requires action and it may be that people who become physically active on a regular basis are simply action-oriented people or "doers." However, I believe that a reasonably high proportion of people are capable of making significant changes in lifestyle. I wouldn't have written this book if I didn't strongly believe this. I have seen countless numbers of college-age students as well as the middle-aged and even the elderly initiate and adhere to exercise programs. So, if I trust my observations, I believe we will continue to see a rise in the percentage of Americans who exercise enough to derive some of the many benefits.

As a physical education teacher with experience teaching and coaching in the public schools, teaching for 15 years at a university, and studying the effects of exercise on people ranging in age from 6 to more than 80 years old, I have learned some valuable tips on how to enhance motivation to exercise. Let me share some with you.

Write down specific fitness and/or performance objectives. Writing down a goal or objective forces you to commit yourself to something definite. Make sure it is realistic. Leave the statement of your objective where it will be seen frequently. I paper clip mine to the front of my exercise diary so I see it daily.

Give your exercise program a fair chance to demonstrate its effects. Measurable gains in some aspects of fitness such as strength and aerobic power can occur in a period of less than 2 weeks. Other fitness components, such as reduction of body fat, take a longer period. At the levels of exercise commonly used by most people, you may not perceive any real changes for 6 to 8 weeks. So, give it time.

I think exercise will have to be performed for several months, however, before it becomes a habit. About 50% of people who start exercise programs drop out within the first

6 months. However, some research data show that the probability of exercise becoming part of one's lifestyle markedly increases once the 6-month period has been surpassed. When you have made exercise a habit, you will feel guilty when you miss a scheduled day of exercise. The ultimate goal is for exercise to be such a basic aspect of your life that you make some time available nearly every day for physical activity. Those of us who are chronic exercisers don't ask ourselves each day "Shall I exercise?" but "When shall I exercise?" or "What shall I do for exercise today?"

Keep an exercise diary. I record all of my exercise sessions in a notebook each day and have done so since I was a senior in high school. There must be some value or reason for doing it because many runners and athletes have done it over the years. Many runners, cyclists, and swimmers like to keep track of the miles they cover each week, month, and year. It does provide a feeling of accomplishment. Logs or diaries for runners are available commercially in most sporting goods stores. They can be used, however, for any activity.

Do something to maintain the habit. Even if time isn't available for your normal-length session, do a miniworkout just to keep the engine tuned and the mind habituated. The important thing is not letting one missed session set a pattern for making it easier to skip the next time you have a busy day. Just the mere act of doing something physical contributes to a sense of accomplishment rather than failure. When out of town at a professional meeting, I jog 2 out of the 3 days or 3 out of the 4 days I'm gone. I do a minicalisthenic routine such as push-ups and sit-ups on the one day I don't jog and add some extra walking to sightsee. After months or years of daily exercise, the body seemingly wants activity of some sort almost daily.

Exercise with other people. This may be as basic a principle of motivation for exercise as exists. The great majority of people who begin an exercise program exercise with other people. Most people, quite honestly, don't need the special exercise equipment in a YMCA or commercial studio to train effectively but exercise is big business because most people seem to need the company of others. While I don't think the "misery loves company" idea holds true for most people who exercise, we are all social animals to some extent. Walking or jogging with a friend is a nice way to make exercise pleasant. It's also a nice way to meet people.

College students where I teach say that the jogging trail and weight room on our campus are the "hot spots"for meeting prospective dates. A number of recent publications indicate that today's young urban professionals consider the jogging trails, racquetball clubs, and tennis clubs the best places to meet the opposite sex. It does sound like a healthier meeting place than the singles' bars of the 1970s.

Exercise to music. Fifteen years ago this idea would have sounded novel to most people. The popularity of aerobic dance is astounding. It seems that nearly every church and school in Omaha serves as an aerobic dance studio in the evenings. Even many businesses become aerobic dance facilities immediately after work. Why the popularity? The music is obviously a major factor.

I always include aerobic dance for one or two activity segments in a fitness course I teach. Female students rate it as the single most popular activity we do, whereas men rate it number two. The men usually have to go through a disinhibition period, which usually lasts until about 10 minutes after they see their professor "let loose." Music of the right sort just makes movement want to happen. The fun thing is that most aerobic dance teachers include a little bit of simple choreography most people can quickly learn. A little bit of dancer is in many of us.

Wear fun exercise clothes. It is fun to wear bright, happy exercise clothes. Today's fashions are a far cry from the old gray sweats we wore when I was in high school and college. Just buying a new pair of running shoes or shorts makes me want to get out and run.

Schedule exercise into your day. You will do this automatically after becoming a chronic exerciser but to start out you will need to do this or the free time to exercise will never be found. Block off the time for exercise on your calendar or schedule and treat it like any other appointment. It may seem selfish at first, but you will get used to it. It makes it a lot easier to tell someone "I have an appointment at that time" than to treat it as something of low priority and let other activities preclude your exercise.

Research on exercise adherence at the famous Aerobic Research Institute in Dallas indicates that people who exercise in the morning miss fewer sessions than those who exercise later in the day. The disadvantage is that the injury rate is higher probably because people may be more hurried early in the day and do not thoroughly warm up. Also, the body temperature is lower in the morning than later in the day, which means that warming up of the connective tissues takes longer.

Include variety in your exercise program. The same type of exercise performed at the same location and at the same time of day is soon going to become monotonous for most people. I have always enjoyed jogging but I vary the type of running I do from season to season. I typically run some road races in the summer and fall. During these months I train differently. I run some fast intervals two or three times a week (an interval workout incorporates alternating fast and slow periods of running such as running 3 minutes at a brisk competitive speed followed by a minute or two of slow jogging to recuperate) and on 1 day each week I will run a relatively long time, about an hour to an hour and a half, at a comfortable pace. On the days in between these training sessions I do a comfortable steady pace run of 30 to 40 minutes. Furthermore, I use three or four different routes and get on a track only once every one or two weeks. So, there can be quite a bit of variation even in something as simple as running.

In the winter I enjoy cross-country skiing when there is adequate snow and I play basketball about twice a week, cycle once or twice a week, and reduce my running to 3 or 4 days a week.

As regards muscular fitness and flexibility, a wide variety of exercises exists to strengthen or stretch any part of the body. A review of chapters 7 and 8 will point this out. I vary weight training exercises about every 2 months purely to keep this aspect of my training challenging and enthusiastic. Most weight trainers and weight lifters do the same. If training doesn't involve a sense of enthusiasm and enjoyment, then it should signal that it is time for a change.

Incorporate household chores into your fitness program. I sometimes substitute cutting the grass for my daily aerobic workout. Trimming hedges by hand without electric clippers could certainly replace a weight training session, as could shoveling snow or raking leaves. I've even heard of people who vacuum and dust the house with great vigor while listening to music. I think that fit people seek ways to *use* their fitness, and many physically active people actually do such chores as mentioned here on top of whatever recreational fitness activity has been done or will be done that day. The fit get fitter and sedentary people continue to fall behind.

Parents, play vigorous games with your children. This is a nice way to enjoy being with your children. It's good for you and your children and the particular benefit may be that your children can see it is normal for adults to play and be physical. Such an attitude may make it easier for your children to be more active, fit, and healthy as adults. I think most parents would find that playing soccer, tag, frisbee, kick the can, and tossing a ball can be high quality time spent with their children. When is the last time you played with your child?

Read reinforcing literature. Some people are difficult to persuade. My brother-in-law used to tease me about my running when our families were together for holidays. He was aware I felt he should exercise because he was overweight and his cholesterol level was too high. I used the best of my psychological ploys for quite a few years trying to get him to start a fitness program but to no avail. What eventually did the trick was giving him a copy of Kenneth Cooper's book on aerobics.

The book summarized all the medical benefits and cited supporting references. This scientific, lay-the-facts-on-the-table approach must have appealed to his engineering background.

I know many runners who have subscribed for years to various running magazines. Many say it is highly motivating to read about the championship marathoners, how they train and eat, and other aspects of their lifestyles. The circulation of *Runner's World* magazine is about a half million so its message must have quite an appeal. As a runner I can attest to its effect on my enthusiasm for running.

A huge number of books, articles and magazines are available on topics related to fitness and health in general. A visit to the library or newsstand may provide something motivational for you.

Include some activities you enjoyed as a youth in your fitness program. I played all the major sports as a youngster and in addition enjoyed a lot of bicycling, climbing trees, sledding, snowball fights, and other activities. It's amazing how much fun all of these activities are. I still love playing catch with my sons, running football pass patterns, and playing two-on-two front yard soccer. Nearly any game you did as a youngster can be played by an adult who warms up properly and uses some restraint. All of your fitness program doesn't have to be tightly structured so that heart rate or repetitions are counted. As a matter of fact, it is rather nice to make some of your exercise spontaneous and unregimented.

Visit a hospital and observe the handicapped in the physical therapy department, cancer clinic, or cardiology department. Think of what it would mean not to be able to move your body in an unrestricted manner. Watch how the physically handicapped struggle to perform basic movements such as moving out of bed, eating, and drinking. Be thankful for the few limitations healthy diabetics have. Think about the value of exercise in your overall diabetic care. Think about the unfortunate diabetics who never really believed retinopathy, neuropathy, and other problems could happen to them.

Fill a knapsack with 20 pounds of sand. Wear the knapsack for an entire day. At the end of the day, evaluate how your feet, knees, and back feel. Imagine doing this every day for the rest of your life. Did you start looking for ways to minimize movement by noontime? Did you change your mind about going to fetch something? Did you ask someone to get that something for you? Can you better understand now how obesity can change a person's life? If you suddenly gained 20 pounds, wouldn't you become less physically active?

Have your total fitness capacity evaluated. Call the physical education department in a nearby college or university. Many such departments do fitness testing for a fee. This is the best place to have a valid and reliable assessment done because they will have the best equipment and best-trained personnel. As a second choice I recommend a YMCA. Most of them can do a good evaluation.

I suggest the testing to simply let you know where you presently stand. If you are unfit, the test results may prompt you to get going. Several surveys regarding fitness indicate that many unfit, sedentary people think they don't need any special exercise, but it's hard to argue with valid test results.

If you believe you are too busy to exercise, think again. Surveys indicate that a higher percentage of professionals such as doctors, professors, lawyers, and dentists exercise than do nonprofessionals. Higher levels of education are clearly associated in nearly every survey with more exercise and better eating habits. If these professionals can find the time, one might well wonder about the time management skills of sedentary people who claim they don't have time to exercise. Read a book or attend a seminar on time management; learn how to "create" the time to exercise.

If you think you are too old or too sick to exercise, think again. There are people confined to wheelchairs who have completed a full marathon (26.2 miles) using just the power of their own arms and shoulders. One young Canadian with cancer ran across Canada in an attempt to raise money for cancer research.

Are you aware that men and women in their 70s have run marathons? Do you realize that many physically active men and women in their 50s, 60s, 70s, and 80s compete in track and field and swimming competitions against people their own age? These examples indicate the importance of attitude in determining what people can or cannot do.

Women, realize that sweating is a natural and normal response to work and sport, and that you will not appear unfeminine because you sweat. To women past age 40 or 50, sweating may be perceived as a noxious, dirty, and unfeminine thing to do, especially in public. Today things are different. The secret is out: Women and girls who sweat are "in"! Look at today's commercials. Note how frequently they include men and women doing strenuous physical activity. Society has officially accepted and now even welcomes the physically active, fit, energetic female.

"I'm too embarrassed to be seen in public bouncing around." There is no reason why your own house can't become your exercise studio. Ride a stationary cycle or briskly walk, march, or dance indoors to music. I doubt that anyone thinks it is humorous or unusual to see anyone outside walking or cycling. A huge percentage of the population of all shapes and sizes is out there, too. You may be surprised that a lot of people may admire you for taking action. Joggers and walkers often salute each other with a wave and a smile even when they don't know each other. It is a sign of respect and encouragement.

Avoid injury. One study showed that 17% of the dropout rate in endurance exercise programs was attributed to injury. Make sure you warm up and cool down properly, and you don't let your enthusiasm carry you into exercise sessions that are too long or too intense. We all have a fatigue and injury point unique to each one of us, so do not try to keep up with others regardless of their age or sex. Exercise must be enjoyable and safe if it is to become a part of your life. Train comfortably and sensibly, and avoid the frustration of soreness and injury.

Offer support to those trying to initiate and sustain an exercise program. A number of studies indicate that family support is a good predictor of those who adhere to exercise programs. This is probably of particular importance in the first several months of activity.

Seek to become positively addicted to exercise. Glasser's book, *Positive Addiction,* discusses how one may become addicted to some positive aspect of life such as exercise. This was discussed in some detail in chapter 10. Some runners are addicted in the sense that they experience withdrawal symptoms such as anxiety, restlessness, and insomnia when they miss a day's run. If being unable to exercise makes you anxious and frustrated a bit, it may represent the inability to practice a sound basic health behavior. It would bother me if I was unable to brush my teeth or wash my hands for 24 hours. However, anything, including exercise, can be overdone. A fairly small amount of exercise, 20 minutes a day, will yield many psychological and physical benefits. You don't have to spend hours at a time to derive the positive effects; as a matter of fact, much of the training effect occurs in the initial 20 minutes of exercise.

Glasser believes that physical activity is likely to become positively addicting if it meets the following criteria:

- It is simple to do and does not require more than a few sessions to become proficient in doing it.
- It can be done alone; you don't have to depend on others in order to do it.
- It can be performed noncompetitively.
- You must believe there is some value for you in doing the activity.
- You can do the activity without criticizing yourself. On this point, Glasser emphasizes that you should not compare yourself to others because this will eventually tend to make you criticize yourself.

Many endurance-type activities meet these criteria. So according to Glasser, it isn't necessary that one jog or run to become positively addicted.

Search for "the sweet spot." John Jerome has written several books about the exhilaration that sometimes occurs when our movements become highly efficient. In the parlance of the tennis player, the "sweet spot" is the region in the center of the strings of the racket where optimal power and control are produced. A unique sound punctuates the occurrence of a "sweet" motion in physical activity. When a baseball player hits the ball squarely in the middle with the middle of the bat, and if all the muscle forces produced at each joint summate in perfect timing, the hit is wonderously powerful. The sound of ball and bat colliding is a "crack" rather than a common "thud." The ball goes far and fast, yet there is a sense that the player didn't really swing all-out.

Every sport has its particular sweet spots that make the movement kinesthetically delicious. The more skilled the athlete or mover, the more frequently the sensation can be created. Yet, even in the elite athlete, the champion, it can't always be produced.

Although I was never an elite athlete, I find it quite fascinating to strive for the "sweet spot" in most of the activities I regularly pursue. Every now and then, I get into a groove in shooting a hook shot in basketball, or a supersmooth glide in cross-country skiing, or a fantastically smooth running form that makes 1 out of 30 days of running a true joy. This quest for kinesthetic delight has become a main focus in most of my sporting activity and I suspect it has for thousands of others. You just can't believe how good it feels unless you have experienced it yourself.

The words of one of our champion female sprinters in the 1984 Olympic games succinctly express the potency of feeling derived from finding the "sweet spot." In a TV interview, she explained that the drudgery of her diligent, daily training was more than compensated by the tremendous feeling she experienced occasionally while sprinting. She compared the feeling to sex but added "only better."

Motivating and Helping the Young Diabetic

Finding out that a youngster of 8, 10, or 12 years is diabetic can be an emotionally traumatic event for a parent. The idea of needles, medication, and careful medical monitoring places quite a burden on parents' shoulders. It isn't too surprising that many parents try to help their child so excessively that the child becomes dependent on the parent for measuring the insulin dosage, administering the shot, sticking the finger, and monitoring other aspects of the diabetic regimen. After a month or two of this the child truly is dependent on the parent. This dependence requires continual care by the parent(s), which feeds the sense of being needed. A vicious cycle such as this, once established, is difficult to break. Neither child nor parent(s) is prone to severing this relationship.

I have seen this relationship develop in several families with a diabetic child. I warn you about it because it usually leads to a psychologically "crippled" individual who learns to use the condition as a crutch. An insulin reaction is produced whenever the child is to work, act independently, or do anything that he or she doesn't really want to do. The phrase "I think I have an insulin reaction" becomes so powerful a tool that the child manipulates the environment. Obviously, the child's emotional and social growth suffer under this influence.

Have the courage to let your child understand that diabetes is a part of his or her daily existence that can only be regulated by himself or herself. The motivation to eat properly, take blood sugar tests, take insulin, and maintain a healthy lifestyle can only be developed if the child fully understands and accepts the condition that he or she is primarily responsible. It's great to praise a child who does these things well, but it takes courage, patience, motivation, and lots of love to see that it *is* done well. The process of creating a largely independent diabetic (independent of parents assuming the responsibility) is no different from the development we wish to see in all aspects of a child's behavior, but with a diabetic child this behavior has to mature much sooner.

appendix A

Additional Reading

The American Diabetes Association (1660 Duke St., P.O. Box 25757, Alexandria, VA 22313) and its state-affiliated organizations have many brief and easy to read pamphlets and leaflets. Most of the pamphlets are free of charge (one copy) and can be mailed to you. Topics include all facets of diabetic management including insulin types, administration of the injection, oral medications, diet, recipes, food exchange lists, exercise, and many other related topics. The ADA also publishes *Diabetes Forecast Magazine*, which provides a wealth of practical information. You receive *Forecast* through membership in the ADA.

Ames Division of Miles Laboratories (1127 Myrtle Street, Elkhart, IN 46515) publishes *Diabetes in the News*, a newspaper about research and new developments in the management of diabetes. The newspaper is free.

Part I: The Basics

American Diabetes Association/American Dietetic Association. (1976). *Exchange lists for meal planning. (Available from the American Diabetes Association, P.O. Box 25757, Alexandria, VA 22313.)*

The American Diabetes Association/American Dietetic Association family cookbook. (1981). Englewood Cliffs, NJ: Prentice-Hall.

Boshell, B.R. (1979). *The diabetic at work and play* (2nd ed.). Springfield, IL: Chas. C. Thomas.

Brothers, M.J. (1976). *Diabetes: The new approach.* New York: Grosset and Dunlap.

Middleton, K., & Hess, M.A. (1978). *The art of cooking for the diabetic.* Englewood Cliffs, NJ: Prentice-Hall.

Nutritive value of foods (Home and Garden Bulletin #72). (April, 1981). Washington, DC: U.S. Government Printing Office.

Peterson, C.M. (1979). *Take charge of your diabetes.* Charles Peterson.

Sussman, K.E., & Metz, R.J.S. (Eds.). (1975). *Diabetes mellitus* (4th ed.). New York: American Diabetes Association.

Part II: Physical Fitness

Cooper, K. (1977). *The aerobics way.* New York: Evans Company.

Katch, F.I., & McArdle, W.D. (1977). *Nutrition and weight control.* Boston: Houghton-Mifflin.

Marley, W.P. (1982). *Health and physical fitness.* Philadelphia: Saunders.

Mayer, J. (1975). *A diet for living.* New York: Pocket Books.

Pollock, M.L., Wilmore, J.H., & Fox, S.M. (1984). *Exercise in health and disease.* Philadelphia: Saunders.

Sharkey, B.J. (1979). *Physiology of fitness.* Champaign, IL: Human Kinetics.

Williams, M.H. (1983). *Nutrition for fitness and sport.* Dubuque, IA: Wm. C. Brown.

Part III: Putting It All Together

Benson, H. (1975). *The relaxation response.* New York: Avon Books.

Bierman, J., & Toohey, B. (1977). *The diabetic's sports and exercise book.* Philadelphia: J.B. Lippincott.

Kivelowitz, T.A. (1981). *Diabetes: A guide to self-management for patients and their families.* Englewood Cliffs, NJ: Prentice-Hall.

Selye, H. (1975). *Stress without distress.* New York: Signet.

appendix B

Diabetic Organizations and Community Resources

National Diabetic Organizations

American Diabetes Association (ADA)
1660 Duke St.
P.O. Box 25757
Alexandria, VA 22313

The ADA publishes a magazine bimonthly called *Diabetes Forecast*. It is filled with practical tips on diabetic care and relates personal experiences of diabetics.

International Diabetes Center
4959 Excelsior Boulevard
Minneapolis, MN 55416

The center offers a variety of inexpensive pamphlets, booklets, and slide sets dealing with various facets of diabetes care.

Joslin Diabetes Foundation, Inc.
One Joslin Place
Boston, MA 02215

> This world famous facility has separate divisions for research, education, and youth. Their efforts involve all facets of diabetes management and research. It is one of eight Diabetes Research and Training Centers designated by the National Institute of Health.

Juvenile Diabetes Foundation (JDF)
60 Madison Avenue
New York, NY 10010-1550

> This organization publishes a quarterly magazine called *Dimension*.

National Diabetes Information Clearinghouse
7910 Woodmont Avenue, Suite 1811
Bethesda, MD 10014

> This organization publishes a list of nutrition information related to diabetic management.

Community Resources

Many communities have local chapters of the ADA and JDF. Even in a state like Nebraska where I live, where only two cities have a population exceeding 100,000, there are 38 local chapters of the ADA. In some communities diabetic clubs have been formed that are not affiliated with the ADA or JDF. Many hospitals have programs for diabetics. They typically emphasize education and socialization with other diabetics. Camps for diabetic children exist in many locales.

Newly diagnosed diabetics or diabetics moving to a new community can use the telephone directory to identify local diabetic groups. A call to a local hospital may also be an efficient way of locating diabetes groups and diabetes medical specialists (nurse educator, podiatrist, exercise physiologist, physical therapist, nutritionist, and others). In most cases, you will be surprised how many sources of information and formal education exist in many communities.

References

Berg, K. (1983). Blood glucose regulation in an insulin-dependent diabetic backpacker. *The Physician and Sportsmedicine,* **11**(12), 103.

Berg, K., Sady, S., Beal, D., Savage, M., & Smith, J. (October, 1983). Developing an elementary school CHD prevention program. *The Physician and Sportsmedicine,* **11**(10), 99-105.

Blackburn, G., & Pavlou, M. (1983). Fad reducing diets: Separating fads from fact. *Contemporary Nutrition,* **8**(7), 1-2.

Caffeine: What it does. (October, 1981). *Consumer Reports,* p. 598.

Gilliam, T., Katch, V., & Thorland, W. (1977). Prevalence of coronary heart disease risk factors in active children, 7-12 years of age. *Medicine and Science in Sports,* **9**, 21-25.

Kostrubala, T. (1976). *The joy of running.* Philadelphia: Lippincott.

Pines, M. (December, 1980). Psychological hardiness: The role of challenge in health. *Psychology Today,* p. 34-35.

Wilmore, J.H. (1986). *Sensible fitness* (pp. 189-191). Champaign, IL: Leisure Press.

Index

Adrenal gland, 159, 168, 186
Adrenaline, 168, 177
Adult-onset diabetes, 15, 16
Aerobic fitness, 49-66
    trainability, 56-58
    program, 130
American Diabetes Association, 247, 251
Appetite
    insulin and, 155-157
    mechanisms, 157-161
    suppressants of, 155

Backpacking, 212-214
Behavior, analysis of factors that affect, 224-227
    health, 228-229
Bench press, 81
Bench stepping, 94
Beta endorphins, 13, 177
Blood sugar
    assessment of, 18-20
    correction plan, 24-26
    importance of, 3-7, 13
    see also Hyperglycemia; Hypoglycemia
Blood vessels, complications of, 4-5
Breath, holding of, 73
Breathing, deep, 180

Caffeine, 186-190
Calories, *see* Energy
Change, in weight training schedule, 74-75
Children, *see* Kids
Cholesterol, 4, 8, 56
Complications of diabetes
    eyes, 4
    heart and blood vessels, 4-5
    immune system, 5
    kidneys, 4
    nerves, 3, 4
Cool-down, 45-47

Diabetes
    complications, 3-5
    components of control, 15-17
    types of, 15-16
Diet, *see* Fad diet; Meals; Nutrition; Weight control
Drugs, and stress, 186-190

Eating, motivational tips for, 229-234; *see also* Meals
Efficiency, work, 191, 194-195
Emergency, supplies in car, 204-205
Energy
    cost of exercise, 29-32
    sources of, 32-35

Environment, effects on exercise, 63-64
Exercise
    contraindications, 73-74
    criteria for a successful session, 65-66
    duration, 56
    effect on insulin and oral medication requirement, 35-36
    energy cost, 29-32
    energy sources during, 32-35
    environmental effects, 63-64
    frequency, 56-57
    intensity, 50-56
    mode, 57
    motivational tips, 234-244
    physician approval, 41-42
    principles of, 41-48
    progression, 60-61
    prolonged, 210-215
    values of, 8-9
    warm-up and cool-down, 45-47
    weight training exercises, 78-96
Eyes, complications of, 4

Fad diets, 140-146
Fat
    content in foods, 148-149
    excess, 122-126
    need for, 122
Flexibility
    how to stretch, 111-113
    importance of, 97-99
    testing and developing, 99-111
Frequency, of exercise, 56-57

Glasser, William, 179, 243
Glucose
    assessment, 18-20
    correction plan, 25-26
    day after extensive exercise, 39
    importance of control, 3-7
Glycemic index, 156-157, 185-186
Glycogen, 9

Half-squat, 92
Heart, complications of, 4
Heart rate
    maximum, 52
    training, 52-53
High blood pressure, 4
Holidays, 216-217
Hyperglycemia, 186
    treatment of, 22, 25-26
Hypoglycemia, 186
    treatment of, 25, 206-208

Identification, 204
Illness, 199-200

Immune system, 5
Inactivity, adjustment to, 209-210
Insulin
    and appetite, 155-157
    capacity to exercise, 37-38
    duration of effect, 22
    injection site, 38-39
    multiple injections, 21-23
    reactions during exercise, 23-25
    staying on schedule, 215
    treatment of insulin reaction, 206-208
    types of, 22
Intensity, of exercise, 50-56

Job, adjustment to, 215
Juvenile-onset diabetes, 15-16

Ketones, 9, 144-145
Ketosis, 9, 26, 144-145
    effects of, 9
    and exercise, 37
    and good diabetic control, 13
    treatment, 208-209
Kids
    and diabetes, 245-246
    and weight training, 76-77
Knee extension, 95-96
Kostrubala, Thaddeus, 176

Lat pull, 86
Lente insulin, 22
Life, philosophy of, 196-197
Load, weight training, 70, 71

Maslow, Abraham, 220
Maturity-onset diabetes, 15-16
Meals
    delayed, 205
    frequency of, 151-153
    restaurant, 205, 233
Medications, 185-190, 202-203
Minirebounding, 64-65
Motivation
    for the young diabetic, 245-246
    principles of, 220-224
    tips for exercise, 234-244
    tips on eating, 229-234
Muscular fitness, 10-11, 77-102
    basic exercises, 78-96
    contraindications, 73-74
    definition, 67
    full range of motion, 68-69
    holding breath, 73
    importance, 67-68
    kids and weight training, 76-77
    periodic change, 74-75

progressive overload, 69
repetitions and load, 70-72
sets, 69
specificity of, 72-73
training principles, 68-75

Nerves, complications of, 3-4
Noradrenaline, 168
Nutrition, and exercise, 138, 145

Obesity, see Weight control
Oral hypoglycemic medication, 11, 215
Overload, progression in, 69
Oxygen uptake, maximum, 50-52

Pelvic tilt, 88
Pregnancy, 214
Prescription
    for aerobic exercise, 51-65
    for weight control, 127-133
Progression, in exercise, 60-61
Pull-ups, 87
Push-ups, 83-84

Rebounding, 64-65
Recipes, see Snacks
Relaxation, muscle, 180-181
Repetitions, in weight training, 70-71
Retinopathy, 4
Rope jumping, 64-65
Rowing motion, 85

Satiety, 157-161
Sets, weight training, 69-70
Shock, insulin, see Hypoglycemia
Site, injection, 38-39
Sitting press, 82
Snacks
    low calorie, 153-155
    while traveling, 204
Stair stepping, 94
Strength
    exercises, 78-96
    training principles, 68-75
    see also Muscular fitness
Stress, 12, 13, 203
    coping techniques, 175-185
    deep breathing, 180
    definition, 166-169
    exercise and, 176-179
    muscle relaxation, 180-183
    philosophy of life, 196-197
    symptoms, 174-175
    visualization, 183

work efficiency, 191, 194-196
yoga stretching, 184-190
Stretching
    exercises, 99-111
    how to, 111-113
    importance of, 97-99
    PNF (proprioceptive neuromuscular facilitation), 111-112
Surgery, 200-201

Tes-Tape, 19
Testing, of flexibility, 99-111
Traveling
    prolonged inactivity while, 209-210
    snack food while, 204
Triglyceride, 4
Trunk curl, 89-90
Trunk rotation, 91
Types of diabetes, 15-16

Urinalysis, 19

Vision, 4
Visualization, 183

Walking, 60
Warm-up, 45-47
Weight control, 9-10
    appetite and satiety mechanisms, 157-161
    appetite suppressants, 155
    carbohydrate vs. fat, 146-150
    causes of obesity, 124-126
    dietary aspects, 148-162
    disadvantages of obesity, 116-121
    exercise and appetite, 134-135
    exercise and nutritional status, 138
    exercise prescription for, 127-133
    fad diets and quick weight loss, 140, 143-146
    frequency of meals, 151
    glycemic index, 156-157
    how much fat is too much?, 122-124
    insulin and appetite, 155
    low calorie, high protein diets, 141
    low calorie snacks, 153
    motivational tips, 229-234
    need for fat, 123
    role of exercise, 126-127
    saunas, body wraps, and other devices, 133-134
    societal standards, 118
    women, 121
Weight training, *see* Muscular fitness
Women, and weight control, 121
Work, efficiency of, 191, 194-196

Yoga, 184-185

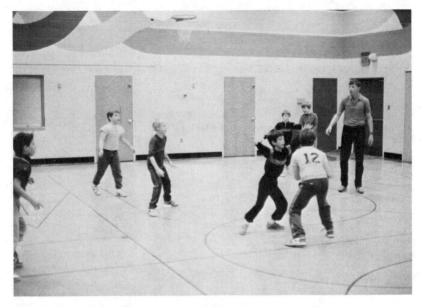

Kris and his third grade basketball team

About the Author

Maintaining good health and an active lifestyle have been two of Kris Berg's primary goals since he was diagnosed as having diabetes at age 12. Kris is now a professor in the School of Health, Physical Education, and Recreation at the University of Nebraska at Omaha where he also is coordinator of the exercise physiology laboratory and university fitness center. He received his EdD in physical education from the University of Missouri. Kris has authored over 50 journal articles on a variety of topics related to sports medicine and exercise physiology and has made hundreds of presentations and workshops on exercise, fitness, stress adaptation, management of diabetes, and sports.

Kris enjoys coaching youth sports, running, cross-country skiing, backpacking, backyard sports, reading, and writing. His wife Carolyn and their sons Eric and Steve share his enthusiasm for maintaining an active lifestyle.